Praise for Yoga 1
Timeless Mind-Body Pra

Transformational, skillful and highly experiential. In *Yoga Meditations* we move beyond yoga as physical posturing and learn the subtle teachings of inner yoga — the way of mind, heart and spirit. Not only does this approach facilitate healing our relationship to ourselves, others and our world, it describes in detail how to fulfill our deepest longing and realize our highest potentials. As a teacher and practitioner for more than 30 years, I am thrilled to finally have such a trustworthy resource to share with my students and my Self. She presents complex teachings of yoga with easy clarity and humor, and then touches us with real stories of her own difficult journey of awakening. Because she has the rare ability to both instruct and inspire, Julie's approach brought me to the real core of yoga — a compassionate awakening to myself as a spiritual being living a human life — and gave me new skills by which to extend that awareness to others.

Christopher Baxter — President AtmaYoga Educational Services

Julie Lusk brings a contemporary look into these ancient teachings. These practices will soothe your soul and soften your heart. I am happy to be a part of this beautiful book.

Lilias Folan — Host of PBS yoga series *Lilias!*

Yoga Meditations offers a wonderful and generous assortment of simple but powerful, eminently practical practices to guide and empower its readers, from beginner to sophisticate.

Belleruth Naparstek — Psychotherapist, author of *Invisible Heroes: Survivors of Trauma and How they Heal* and creator of Health Journeys guided imagery

Finding the words to guide students into an experience of the formless is always a challenge. *Yoga Meditations* provides a wide range of language and an array of approaches that will inform and inspire any teacher of yoga and meditation.

Jonathan Foust — President Emeritus, Kripalu Center for Yoga and Health

An abundant treasure of ideas for those who work in the realms of guided imagery, hypnotherapy, trance induction, yoga, meditation, healing, and chakra work. A gift to the faculties of human imagination.

Anodea Judith — author of *Wheels of Life, Eastern Body: Western Mind*

This book is user friendly.

Brenda deMartine — Wellness Educator and Yoga Teacher

Yoga Meditations

Timeless Mind-Body Practices for Awakening

Julie Lusk, M.Ed, RYT

Whole Person Associates
Duluth, Minnesota

Whole Person Associates
210 West Michigan Street
Duluth, MN 55802-1908
800-247-6789

Yoga Meditations
Timeless Mind-Body Practices for Awakening

Printed in the United States of America

10 9 8 7 6 5 4 3 2 1

ISBN 1-57025-216-5

Library of Congress Control Number: 2005922849

Table of Contents

Dedication and Acknowledgements

Yoga Meditations: Timeless Mind-Body Practices for Awakening is dedicated to the two most important men in my life: my beloved husband, Dave, and my brother, Tom Tapin.

Dave is my earth angel. He keeps me grounded and gives me extraordinary love and support. He is my best friend and always believes in me. Dave was always willing to interrupt whatever he was doing and lend his help by allowing me to try a variety of mind-body practices with him. This was especially valuable because he is not the yoga meditation type. He even tried the yoga postures. I knew that if it worked for him, it worked. Dave drew the illustrations when my original plan fell through.

Tom is my celestial angel. He lived a remarkable life that often seemed enchanted. His life took him around the globe as he explored worldly as well as spiritual frontiers. His friendships were strong, important, and spanned the world. He was energetic, spirited, generous, friendly, smart, funny, and handsome. We were incredibly blessed to be a brother and sister with souls that connected so deeply. In November 2003, Tom died unexpectedly after a very brief illness while he was living and working in Venezuela. My heart broke. Over the next four months, his life was honored and celebrated with memorials in Venezuela, California, and finally in Ohio. These tributes gave us a chance to remember his life and say good-bye for now. It also kept my intense grief and strong emotions right on the surface.

All my life, I've sought to be of service and to use my talents in useful ways. More than ever before, I prayed for guidance and opportunities to be positive and productive. The Monday following Tom's final Mass a call came from Whole Person Associates asking me to write this book. The timing was heaven sent. This project came to me right when I needed it most. In fact, I had been floating this book idea for over two years and couldn't understand why it was so elusive. Now as I look back, I realize that it had been developing all along. What I thought of as independent projects were really gems that were finally being strung together into a garland. I was on my path all along. I just didn't know it. My faith renewed.

The practices within *Yoga Meditations* were my salvation, anchoring me with soft strength and giving me much needed courage and openness to heal my wounded and grieving heart. I don't know how I would have managed without the spacious awareness cultivated by mindfulness, the practice of being in the present moment, the breathwork that could either calm or energize me, knowing how to transform unwanted thoughts and feelings with Tonglen and Pratipaksha Bhavana, and being able to profoundly rest through the relaxation practices. Yoga's ancient and contemporary wisdom teachings and prayers enlarged my perspective and opened and soothed my heart and soul. Nearly every night of the week, the students in my yoga classes inspired and supported me as I shared hatha yoga with them. God bless every one of them.

Years of actively practicing moment-to-moment awareness while doing hatha yoga rewarded me by allowing me to naturally live in the moment while off my mat and meditation cushion. The focused awareness I was able to maintain let me notice the inspiring miracles that were happening all around me and gave me the mental and emotional space needed to embrace the mystery of it all. Sparkling joy, outrageous beauty, inner strength, and deep faith were always found tucked within the sadness.

The ancient yoga masters are right: The experience of yoga is profoundly healing and revealing. I am forever thankful.

I offer my heartfelt gratitude to so many along my path. Christopher Baxter was steadfast in his perspective and help with reviewing *Yoga Meditations*. His insights, humor and help were invaluable.

Lilias Folan, Sudhir Jonathan Foust, Nischala Joy Devi, Lynne Greene, Charles MacInerney, Don Tubesing, Sally Kempton, and Christopher Baxter graciously and willing shared transcripts of their meditations for inclusion in this book. Their contributions enrich and magnify the scope of this work immeasurably.

Anodea Judith, Laurie Moon, Julia Young, Janet Chahrour, Nancy Spence, Julie Isphording, Georg Feurstein, Mark Weisberg, and Connie and Vince Lasorso each came to my rescue when I got stuck when trying to capture concepts that are beyond words.

My yoga teachers light my way. I am especially grateful to Joe Panoor, Tracey Rich, Ganga White, Lilias Folan, Ram Dass, Nischala Joy Devi, Christopher Baxter, and Barb Black.

Belleruth Naparstek has taught me much about guided imagery through her books, recordings, website and friendship. Her leadership in medically-related guided imagery has benefited countless people.

Noreen Wessling, Linda McCachran-Brown, Albert Bollinger, Beth

Coulson, Debbie Jackson, Janet Levy, Val Shanks, Cathy Barney, Renee Groenemann, Beth Owens, Laurie Moon, Dan Roche, Greg Mayers, Hildy Getz, Edna Henning, Pat Sollinger, Jane Smith, and Linda Cox are my meditation sisters and brothers. We have explored, questioned, laughed, cried, and supported one another in our meditation practice and in our lives.

Karen Sawyer, Beth Owens, Dina Morelli, Judy Fulop, Diana Mauriello, Micki Wilcox, Janet Reckers Picciano, Mark Skelton, Bharat Lindemood, Michael Baugh, Bob Letscher, Carol Prentice, Ujjayi Bob Clark, and John Flower are dear friends who have been especially helpful and encouraging during this passage of this amazing journey.

Diane Utaski, Kris Gentry, Gayle Schubert, Karen Landrum, Julie Keefe, Karen Popham, Linda Wallace, Nancy Radtke, BevySue Hammons, Marianne Lang, Judie Kelly, and Susan Winter Ward are a few of my yoga buddies. In their own way, each was most helpful. Thank you from my heart.

Many thanks to the Cincinnati Yoga Teachers Association, especially Pooja Malhotra for the Sanskrit lessons.

This book would not have been possible without the expertise and friendship of Carlene Sippola, Susan Rubendall, and Joy Dey at Whole Person Associates. Through CardplusCD, Jean Peters and Tom Laskey have encouraged and supported me in recording many of these guided relaxation and imagery practices, including the ones in this book.

Above all, my love and appreciation stream out to my mom and dad, Angie and Tom, to my sister, Mary Noel Nichols, and her remarkable family, and return full circle to my husband, Dave, and my brother, Tom.

Introduction

Those who go to the very depths of meditation and
realize the Self within the heart
stand firm, grow rich,
gather a family around them,
and receive the love of all.
— Taittiriya Upanishad II. 6.1

The goal of yoga,
union with the Spirit,
can only be known through experience,
not through simply learning or relying
on understanding with the mind.
— Upanishads.

No effort is wasted and
no gain is ever lost when on this path;
even a little practice
will shelter you from sorrow
and protect you from the greatest fear.
— Bhagavad Gita 2.40

Yoga Teacher Student Prayer

OM saha navavatu	May we be protected together.
saha nau bhunaktu	May we be nourished together.
saha viryam karavavahai	May we create strength
tejasvi navadhitam astu	among one another.
ma vidvishavahai	May there be no enmity between us.
OM shanti shanti shanti	Om peace, peace, peace.

For yogis, it comes as no surprise when researchers report that the mind and body are one. This has been a tenet of yoga since ancient times. In modern times, scientists and medical professionals are confirming this belief through rigorous studies and research. They report that meditation, controlled breathing, deep relaxation, and directed, guided imagery can boost the immune system, alter blood pressure, decrease pain and help with problems such as infertility and insomnia. These practices can help people cope with and recover from unpleasant medical procedures as well as the effects of stress from daily living. It is also being verified that each emotion has a distinct biochemical signature that affects mental and physical health.

This book presents a variety of mind-body practices based on yoga. Guided relaxation exercises, breathing practices, guided imagery, affirmations, and meditations are included. You will learn to distinguish the similarities, differences, uses, and benefits for each. Most important, you will be able to practice them yourself as well as lead others through guided exercises.

The exercises identified as "practices" are intended for individual use. With a few modifications, they can also be used to guide others.

Those that use the term "guided" are designed for teachers, workshop leaders, and helping professionals to use in leading others through the experiences in classes and in group or private sessions. They can be modified to suit various needs. For example, many can be shortened, combined with others, or used to spark the leader's own creative experience.

To get the full benefit from these experiences, select one of these options:

1. Have someone softly and slowly read the instructions to you;
2. Familiarize yourself with the instructions and proceed on your own;
3. Make an audio recording to play back for personal use.

Follow the directions as you read through the instructions. The ellipses (…) used throughout the exercises indicate a brief pause.

The most important thing is to practice!

Mind-Body Connection

The mind and body are intimately and ultimately linked as one. There is no separation. What is thought or felt resonates throughout the body, moment by moment, through a biochemical reaction. This reaction is either life and health enhancing or defeating.

The positive aspects of this connection contribute to:

- The ability to recognize one's life purpose and accomplish life dreams and goals
- Feelings of contentment
- A life that is in balance
- Physical, emotional, and mental well-being
- An awakened spirit
- Peace and happiness

The mind-body connection, when ignored, can:

- Undermine one's health physically, mentally, and emotionally
- Create negativity
- Block the flow of creative and healing energy
- Contribute to illness, injuries and disease
- Cause unhappiness and dissatisfaction

Transformational tools that activate and assist the development of a life-enhancing mind-body connection include:

- Focused breathing practices
- Guided relaxation
- Guided imagery and creative visualization
- Affirmations
- Meditation
- Mind-body fitness modalities, such as yoga and tai chi
- Honest expression and congruence of thoughts, feelings, and actions

The following table describes the similarities and differences associated with each of the mind-body techniques presented in *Yoga Meditations: Timeless Mind-Body Practices for Awakening*. The lines between many of the practices are subtle, but each has its own distinct purpose.

Distinctions	Breathing Practices	Guided Relaxation (Yoga Nidra)	Guided Imagery	Affirmations	Meditation
Description	Consciously breathing fully and completely. Various breathing techniques and patterns can be used. Body based.	Purposefully and constructively releasing tension and relaxing the body, mind, emotions and spirit. Body based.	Intentional and useful daydreaming that is multi-sensory and practiced while in a relaxed state. Mind/emotion based.	Repeating brief, uplifting statements that are said in the present tense. Mind/emotion based.	Focusing the mind and emotions. Settling the mind into stillness. Experience the spirit directly. Non-mental and/or mental
Benefits	Oxygenates the body. Detoxifies the system. Calms the nerves. Clears the mind. Prelude to relaxation, guided imagery and meditation.	Relaxes the body, mind, emotions and spirit. Can help various medical conditions.	Can heal the body of various ailments. Increases intuition. Fosters insight. For enjoyment and relaxation.	Increases inner strength and energy. Counteracts negative thoughts and feelings.	Nurtures the spirit. Calms the mind and emotions. Provides mental clarity and perspective. Can help various medical conditions.
Suggestions for practice	Breathing is a complete practice on its own. It can be practiced with guided relaxation, affirmations, imagery, and meditation.	Guided relaxation is a complete practice on its own. It can be practiced with breathing, affirmations, and imagery.	Imagery is less effective if it is done without using breathing or guided relaxation prior to it for centering and relaxing the body and mind.	Affirmations can be said by themselves. Breathing and guided relaxation can be added to strengthen the impact. Affirmations can be added to a meditation.	Meditation is usually practiced by itself. Breathing is often done prior to meditation as a centering devise or as a meditation practice.

Distinctions	Breathing Practices	Guided Relaxation (Yoga Nidra)	Guided Imagery	Affirmations	Meditation
Solo or with others	Breathing can be done solo or in a group led by a person or with a recording.	Guided relaxation is done in a group with a leader, or with a recording. With practice, it can be done solo.	Guided imagery is done in a group with a leader, or with a recording. With practice, it can be done solo	Affirmations are usually done solo. Sometimes with others	Meditation is usually done solo. It can also be guided by a group leader or with a recording.
Physical Position Details are described in the following section.	Lying on a carpet or a mat. Sitting on a straight chair or on the floor.	Usually lying, sometimes sitting in a comfortable chair.	Usually lying, sometimes sitting in a comfortable chair.	Anytime, anywhere.	Sitting on a straight chair or floor with a meditation cushion. Walking.
Optimal time frame As with everything, regular practice yields the best results.	24/7 Breathe fully and consciously for brief intervals on a regular basis. Practice mindfully and regularly for 5 or more minutes at a time.	20 to 30-minute segments are optimal.	10 to 30 minutes per session.	Repeat affirmations regularly and often. Most take less than a minute.	20 or so minutes per session. Practice a minimum of once per day, twice per day when possible.

Prelude to Guided Imagery and Meditation

The cornerstone of all guided imagery and meditation is the ability to relax the body, clear the mind, and settle the emotions. Unfortunately, many people assume that taking the time for relaxation and centering is optional or a waste of time and omit it. Instead they go right to the method and then wonder why they are so distracted.

No one would consider stopping a car going fifty-five miles per hour by pulling the key out of the ignition. In effect, this is what is attempted when the proper preparations are not undertaken prior to guided imagery and meditation. To stop a car, you must first take your foot off the gas, apply it to the brake, wait for the car to stop, take the transmission out of gear, and then remove the key.

Similarly, steps must be taken to prepare the body, mind, and emotions for guided imagery and meditation. For instance, it is important to prepare the body with an appropriate posture and to consciously relax the muscles, joints, and nerves.

It is equally important to prepare the mind and emotions. Slow, deep breathing focuses attention and promotes concentration. Having a focal point for concentration is essential and so is knowing how to handle all sorts of distractions. After all, the mind assumes its job is to think and comment on everything that happens, not to mention its tendency to jump from one subject to another. In reality, cultivating present-moment awareness without getting lost in or identifying with our thoughts is a primary goal of meditation. Concentration on the images, sensations, and affirmations of mindfulness techniques is at the core of those practices.

Guided relaxation, breathwork, and imagery may be done effectively either sitting or lying down. However, sitting upright is an important ingredient for meditation. Recommendations for lying and sitting in each exercise are provided to maximize effectiveness. A person's temperament and preferences will guide the choice of technique. Fortunately, there are a variety of approaches based on the body, breath or mind. Examples of each approach are provided below. Plan to spend a minimum of five minutes prior to practicing a guided imagery or meditation session to fully prepare yourself for the practice. Take more time if necessary. For the best experience possible, use these approaches sincerely, with patience, compassion, and perseverance.

Body-based

Deep relaxation can be accomplished by tensing and releasing muscles using a relaxation exercise or by deepening and slowing the breath while letting go of all physical, mental, and emotional tension. A relaxed state can also be attained by systematically giving the feet, legs, hips, torso, shoulders, arms, and face permission to release tension. Remember that being able to relax is the foundation for all guided visualization exercises. While relaxation can be done by itself, visualizations should always be preceded with a relaxation exercise.

Breathing-based

Breathwork offers a portable paradise when it is used properly. Breathing slowly, smoothly, and evenly is optimal. Allowing the exhalation to naturally become longer than the inhalation is deeply relaxing and slows the heartbeat. The mind calms when it focuses on the present moment awareness of each breath.

Mind-based

Focusing the mind on a sound, thought, word, image, or phrase for a designated amount of time is calming. Instead of being distracted, the mind is trained to concentrate on the moment at hand. This is done by choosing something to focus on, noticing when the mind wanders, and gently bringing attention back to the focal point.

Shavasana (shah-VAH-sah-nah)
Proper Supine Position for Relaxation and Guided Imagery

The optimal position for guided relaxation and imagery is called Shavasana (sponge or corpse pose) in yoga. Shavasana is done lying down on a firm, flat surface, such as a carpeted floor or mat. A sofa or bed can be used; however, you risk falling asleep if it is too comfortable.

Here are the specifics:

Lie down on a carpeted floor or mat. Feel free to cover yourself with a blanket for warmth and comfort.

Start with a nice big stretch. Next, take in a deep breath and sigh it out through an open mouth.

Close your eyes or keep them barely open. An eye pillow or folded washcloth placed over the eyes helps the brain and body relax further.

Place your legs straight out with your heels twelve to twenty-four inches apart. Find a good distance for your feet so that your hips and back can relax. If your back is uncomfortable, bend your knees and lean them against each other with your feet placed on the floor below them. Start by placing your feet wider than your hips, and notice if it feels comfortable and stable. If not, adjust the placement of your feet and knees. An alternative is to place a sturdy pillow or bolster under your knees. Take the time you need to find the optimal position for your comfort.

Lift your hips up slightly and place them back down so they feel supported and your weight is evenly distributed.

Draw your shoulders downward by gently lowering them toward your ears. Snuggle and tuck them in so they rest comfortably beneath you.

Stretch your arms out and away from your sides in a position of ease. Place your palms face up and notice how this feels to you. If you prefer, turn your palms down or place them on your body.

It is important to preserve the natural arch at the back of your neck. To do so, rest the back of your head on the floor and make sure that neither your forehead nor chin is higher than the other. You may use a small pillow under your head, or roll up a small towel and place it under your neck.

Let your awareness roam around your body to become aware of any area that may be uncomfortable and take the time needed to adjust your clothing and your posture so you are totally at ease.

Sitting for Guided Breathing and Meditation

> *With upright body, head, and neck,*
> *lead the mind and its powers into your heart.*
> —Upanishads

Posture plays a significant role in meditation practice. It is important to find a way of sitting that allows your spine to be upright yet not rigid. Doing so enables your energy to flow naturally and your meditation to deepen. While slouching might feel more familiar in the beginning, it will inevitably tire your back, and your hips and shoulders will ache. If your sitting posture is uncomfortable, your awareness will be drawn to these aches and pains instead of inward for meditation. A regular yoga practice helps prevent this by increasing flexibility, strength, and awareness.

It is perfectly acceptable to sit on a chair for meditation. If this is your preference, choose one that has a firm seat — not an easy chair. Place both feet parallel on the floor without crossing your legs or feet. Adjust the height of your chair so your feet rest on the floor and your knees are slightly below your hips. If your chair seat is too high or your legs are too short for comfort, place something under your feet. On the other hand, it is preferable to use an easy chair for guided relaxation and breathing,

Sitting on the floor is another option. Once again, it is important to sit in a way that keeps your back straight but not stiff. Be certain that your lower back maintains its natural, soft curve and does not cave in or become rounded. It is also important that your knees are not sticking up in the air. Instead, your knees should be below the level of the top of your hips.

You can choose from several ways of sitting on the floor. For example, try sitting on a folded blanket or on a meditation bench or meditation cushion. Cross your legs in front of you with one foot placed in front of the other or with your feet tucked under the opposite thigh. Another alternative is to kneel with a firm cushion under your hips and between your legs. Position your legs and feet behind you and out to each side of the cushion.

Whether you are sitting on a chair or on the floor, center your weight primarily upon your sitz bones, located at the very base of your pelvis. Doing so will give you a strong base of support, help maintain the natural curves of your spine, keep you aware and alert, and encourage the flow of energy. Resist the tendency to roll back and sit on your tailbone or sacrum. This will cause you to slouch and round your back, and it will dampen your energy and awareness.

Next, make sure your pelvis is level, not tipping either backward or forward. This will help align your spine and improve your energy. Draw your shoulders up toward your ears, circle them back, and then slide your shoulder blades down your back.

In addition, slightly lift your sternum to tone your abdominal muscles, support your low back, and give more room for your heart and lungs to work.

Next, position your chin so that it is parallel to the floor or tipped slightly downward. This will help release neck tension and will enable better communication to take place between your brain and body. Unclench your teeth, soften your palate, and relax your tongue, allowing it to rest softly inside your mouth.

Rest your hands on your lap. There are several options for positioning your hands. Try out each one and then decide for yourself which feels most comfortable to you. First, try cupping one hand in the other, placing the tips of your thumbs together. Second, try resting one hand on each knee. If your palms are up, you are more likely to feel more open and aware; whereas you may feel calmer if your palms face downward.

Notice how it feels to bring the pads of your thumb and index finger together. The thumb represents your higher self and your first finger represents your individual self. Touching them together represents the unification of your personal and universal self. It is fine for your thumb and fingers to remain apart. Go for what feels right to you. Let your body awareness decide instead of your mind.

Finally, return your awareness back to your sitz bones and settle your weight downward while gently lengthening your spine by lightly lifting your sternum and the crown of your head upward. Sitting should feel natural, steady and comfortable.

Guidelines for Practicing Deep Relaxation and Guided Imagery

Guided imagery, sometimes called guided visualization, is healing to the mind, body, emotions and spirit. Everyone is different and will experience guided imagery uniquely. These individual differences should be encouraged, honored, and cherished. Some people "see" vivid scenes, colors, and images, while others are receptive to their feelings and can sense the images. Being sensitive to sounds is another way to experience imagery. This is why a combination of sights, sounds, smells, and feelings should be incorporated into all guided imagery exercises. With practice, it is quite possible to expand the range of personal awareness to include more senses.

Basics for Group Leaders Leading Guided Relaxation, Imagery, and Meditations

Setting the Mood
Working with deep relaxation and guided imagery is very powerful so please act responsibly. Don't be tempted to use scripts and themes in which you lack training or to work in areas that are unfamiliar to you. Use your best judgment when selecting a guided meditation and always be ethical.

The Right Atmosphere
For deep relaxation and guided imagery, choose a room that has a carpeted floor for lying down or comfortable chairs.

Straight-backed chairs are best for meditation and most breathing practices. Sitting on the floor on a meditation cushion, called a zafu, is another option.

Close the door and shut the windows to block out noise. Adjust the thermostat so the room is warm and comfortable.

Dim the lights to create a relaxing environment. This blocks out visual distractions, enhancing people's ability to relax. If the lights can't be controlled to your satisfaction, bring along a lamp or night-lights. Candles can be used, as long as you are cautious about safety.

Props often enhance comfort when people are lying down. They may need a bolster or a firm pillow under their legs for back comfort; an eye pillow to soothe their eyes and brain; rolled towels to place under their head, neck, or other areas for support; or a blanket for warmth.

Selecting Music
Wisely select music to fit the theme of the experience as well as the people involved. Choose music without lyrics that has simple and flowing melodies. Complex harmonies may be counterproductive. Music is not always necessary and can be omitted, but if you use it, cue it up in advance.

Do not assume that the type of music you find relaxing will be relaxing to others. A person's ability to relax to music is usually related to how well the person likes it. Check it out. Ask for feedback.

Try using sounds from nature like ocean waves. Experiment with music composed for relaxation to find selections that are suitable. Classical music may be effective, especially movements marked largo or adagio. These markings indicate a slow and relaxed tempo.

Adjust the volume so it doesn't overshadow your voice. Music that is too soft, however, may cause your listeners to strain to hear it.

Using Your Voice
Speak in a calm, comforting, and steady manner. Let your voice flow smoothly and somewhat monotonously, but never whisper.

Start with your voice at a volume that can be easily heard. As the guided meditation progresses, begin speaking at a softer volume and tone. Remember, as a person relaxes, hearing acuity increases. Bring your voice up when suggesting tension and bring it down when suggesting relaxation. Return to an easily heard volume near the end of the guided meditation. This will help participants become alert again.

Invite participants to give a hand signal if you cannot be heard. Advise people with hearing difficulties to sit near to you.

Pacing Yourself
Begin at a conversational pace and slow down as relaxation progresses. Take your time and don't rush. Tape yourself to help you improve your volume and tone, pace and timing.

Watch participants carefully to be sure you are giving them time to follow your instructions. For instance, if you suggest that participants wiggle their toes, watch them do so; watch them stop wiggling; and then go on. Sometimes, you will have to repeat instructions if you see that people are not following you.

Preparing the Group or Individual
It is vital to start with a relaxation exercise before doing guided imagery. This helps aid relaxation and enhances concentration. Being physically relaxed reduces anxiety and helps the creative and imaginative "right brain" become active and alert while diminishing the effects of the logical and analytical "left brain."

Before starting, give a brief explanation of the type of imagery to be used and ask if there is anyone who has an objection. Be prepared to change your plans. It is also important to let participants know that they may change images in any way they wish.

It is normal for people to follow you for a while, then tune you out and go into their own imagination. They will usually tune back in later on. If they are made aware of this in advance, they won't feel as if they are "failing." Imagery is most effective when it comes from one's own imagination.

Always draw the relaxation to a close and help participants make the transition back to the present. Bring the participants' attention back to the room by asking them to visualize their surroundings and bring their attention back to their bodies by asking them to stretch and breathe consciously. Repeat these instructions in a louder voice if someone does not begin to move around and stretch at the end of a guided meditation.

Caution
Don't ever force people to participate in anything that may be uncomfortable for them. Give ample permission for everyone to only do things that feel safe. Tell them that if something seems threatening, they can change the image to something that feels right, or they can stop, stretch, and open their eyes.

Handling Distractions
Whenever possible, prevent distractions by closing the door and windows, etc. When unanticipated sounds, such as a noisy air conditioner or a loud conversation in an adjoining room occur, try speaking louder. Use shorter phrases and fewer pauses, or incorporate the sounds into the experience.

Occasionally participants fall asleep and sometimes snore. Once again, plan ahead. Remind people before starting that if they have a tendency to fall asleep or are really tired, to either sit for the experience or keep their eyes slightly open. If someone falls asleep and may be distracting others, raise your voice a bit as this might wake them up. If that doesn't work, quietly walk over and whisper their name or gently nudge their foot. Be sure to let people know in advance that this may happen to them.

Processing The Experience
Add to the richness of the guided meditations by asking participants to share their experiences with others afterwards. This works best if you create an atmosphere of trust. Ask the group open-ended questions that relate to the theme of the exercise. Be accepting and empathetic towards everyone. Respect everyone's comments and never be judgmental or critical.

Sanskrit Pronunciation Guide

Each vowel has a short form and a long form. The long form is pronounced twice as long. A bar is used for the long vowels.

a as in up

ā as in father

i as in give, pin

ī as in easy (held longer)

u as in put

ū as in rule, cool

e as in may

ai as in aisle

o as in go, yoga

au as in cow

Consonants are generally pronounced as in English. However, the following consonants are pronounced with a slight "h" sound. These consonants are B, C, D, G, J, K, P, and T. For example the C is pronounced like ch as in church. The sound of T is as a th as in hothouse and not as in breathe.

Sanskrit Word Guide

    Apana = ah-PAH-nah

    Asana = AH-sah-nah

    Bandha = BAHN-da

    Bhagavad Gita = BHAG -ah -vad GEE-tah

    Chakra = CHA-krah (as in chocolate and rah for chocolate)

  Chakras named from the first to the seventh chakra

      Muladhara = MOOL-ah-dah-ra

      Svadhisthana = SVAH-dees-tah-nah

      Manipura = MAH-nee-poor-ah

      Anahata = AH-nah-hot-ta

      Vissudha = vizh-SHOE-dah

Ajna = AAHJ-nah

Sahasrara = SAH-has-rar-ah

Names for yoga postures for the chakras from the first to the seventh

Child / Garbasana or Balasana = gar-BAH-sah-nah or
bahl-AH-sah-nah

Cat Pose / Bidalasana = bee-doll-AH-sah-nah

Boat / Navasana = nah-VAH- sah-nah

Bridge / Setu Bandhasana = SAY-too bhan-DAH-sah-nah

Supported Fish / Matsyasana = mahtz-YAH-sah-nah

Spinal Twist / Matysendrasana = mahtz-yen-DRAH-sah-nah

Yoga Seal / Yoga Mudra = Yoga MOO-drah

Dharana = DAH-ra-nah

Dhyana = dee-YAH-nah

Dirgha = DEAR-gah

Hari Om = hah-ree OM

Ida = EE-dah

Kapalabhati = KAH-pah-lah-BAH-tee

Koshas in their order

Maya-kosha = MY-ah- KOH-shah

Anna-maya-kosha = AH-nah

Prana- maya-kosha = PRAH-nah

Mano-maya-kosha = MAH-no

Vijnana-maya-kosha = veej-NAH-nah

Ananda – maya-kosha = ah-NAHN-dah

Mudra = MOO-drah

Nadis = NAH-deez

Nadi Shodhana = NAH-dee SHOW-dah-nah

Namaste = nah-mah-STAY

Nidra = NEE-drah

Om Namah Shivaya = OM na-MAH she-VI-yah

Patanjali = pah-TAHN-jah-lee

Pingala = pin-GAH-lah

Pradipika= prah-DEE-pee-kah

Prana = PRAH-nah

Pranayama = PRAH-nah-ya-mah

Pratipaksha Bhahvanah = prah-TEE-pak-shah Bhah-van-ah

Pratyahara = PRAH-tyah-HAH-rah or prat-ya-HAR-ah

Samadhi = sah-MAH-dee

Shanti = SHAN - tee

Sushumna = sue-SHOOM-nah

Trā taka = TRAH- tahk

Ujjayi = oo-JAH-yee

Upanishad = oo-PAH-nee-shad

Yoga Sutra = Yoga Sue-tra

Guided Relaxation: Still Yoga

Yoga is the settling of the mind into stillness.
Our essential nature is usually overshadowed by mental activity.
The five types of mental activity are understanding,
misunderstanding, imagination, sleep and memory.
They may or may not cause suffering.
—Yoga Sutra 1.2, 1.4-6

Stillness. What a treasure in a world that moves at lightening fast speed. Thankfully, there is an ongoing place in each of us that is an unending reservoir of inner strength and stillness. The purpose of yoga and practices like it is to uncover this powerful core and to use it as a solid platform from which to encounter the world and experience life.

Settling mental activity by actively becoming relaxed and centered is an easy starting point for discovering inner peace; it is also the foundation for most mind-body practices. It actively increases our capacity to calm the mind, soothe the emotions, and open the heart.

Practice the following exercises until you become comfortable with them. Each uses a different technique and will enable you to experience relaxation on many levels. Refer to the directions on Shavasana in the introduction to learn the most effective way of lying down for relaxation. Use these practices on their own or combine them with another mind-body practice.

Sinking into Sensation: Here and Now (15 or more minutes)

Squeeze Stress Away (15 minutes)

Breathe, Relax, Feel, Watch, and Allow Meditation (15 to 20 minutes)

Warm Hands (5 to10 minutes)

Complete Relaxation with Yoga Nidra (20 to 30 minutes)

Affirmations for Energy, Strength and Inner Vitality (15 minutes)

Sinking into Sensation: Here and Now

Guided Relaxation

Time: 15 or more minutes

Summary: Physical sensations are the silent language from within our-selves. Softly focusing on what is being felt, sensed, and experienced in the moment leads to an open and ongoing experience of moment-to-moment wakefulness. This essential yet simple awareness exercise guides this powerful process. It is easy to learn and can be used daily for enhancing awareness and mindfulness.

Settle yourself in a comfortable chair or on a mat on the floor. Take a big breath in through your nose ... and sigh it out through your open mouth ... Again, take a big breath in ... and sigh it out. Take notice of how it feels to let your breath release with a sigh.

Close your eyes if they are open ... Can you feel where your eyelids touch?

Notice the surface you are sitting or lying on ... Become aware of where your body meets this surface ... Notice where it feels soft ... where it feels hard ... where there is space.

Treat yourself to a wonderful stretch ... stretch your arms ... your legs ... your back and shoulders ... simply stretch however you would like ... and enjoy your stretch thoroughly.

Pause.

Again, take another full breath in ... and sigh it out.

Allow your body to become still ... settling down, more and more. This is a time for you to experience the inner world of sensations ... the silent language from within ... It will anchor you in the safety of moment-to-moment awareness.

First, listen to the sounds in the room *(name some sounds as they occur — music, the hum of a heater, distant traffic, etc.)* Let each sound come and go ... without resisting it ... or trying to grasp it. ... simply notice the sounds as they occur.

Now, become aware of the clothes against your body . . . and the air on your skin . . . and the back of your body as it rests into what's beneath you.

At any time, feel free to move around . . . and adjust your clothing so you feel as comfortable as you possibly can.

Call to mind what you've been preoccupied with lately . . . Acknowledge what has been on your mind . . . and now, bring your attention to right here, right now . . . letting go of thoughts of the past . . . and of the future.

Become aware of your physical presence . . . your body . . . Let your attention become like a search light . . . and become more and more aware of your physical presence, just as you are.

Pause.

Bring your attention to your energy level . . . become more and more aware of how you feel right now . . . Do you feel tired and washed out? . . . Are you full of pep . . . or somewhere in between? . . . Don't bother to label or name it; it's not important . . . instead, simply sense your energy level just as it is . . . without judgment whatsoever.

Now direct your awareness inside your body and feel it from within. Send your attention to your lower legs . . . Can you feel the life force in your lower legs? This is your subtle energy field. Practice focusing your attention on the sensations in your lower legs. What does it feel like? Do you notice strong sensations or hardly any at all? Feel it instead of thinking about it . . . Let go of the commentary, the judgments, and the mind chatter, and be aware of the sensations in your lower legs.

Now, notice the life force in your knees and upper legs. Once again, instead of labeling and thinking about it, feel the sensations, or perhaps the lack of sensations that are now present in your upper legs.

Can you maintain your awareness throughout your lower and upper legs at the same time?

When your mind starts to lose its focus, kindly bring your awareness back into your body to experience awareness without thinking . . . Be patient. With practice this gets easier and easier.

Bring your awareness to your torso and focus your attention in and around your abdomen, allowing your attention to dwell on the sensations and feelings that are occurring in your abdomen right now . . . Notice if the sensations shift around or if they seem stable . . . Just notice what is happening in your abdomen right now.

Draw your attention into your heart and lungs and become more and more conscious of the feelings and sensations around your heart and lungs.

If thoughts arise, label it thinking and guide your awareness back inside to the sensations that are present.

Now your attention spreads into your shoulders…and arms…and eventually cascades into your hands…Gently hold your attention on your shoulders…arms…and hands.

From here, notice the sensations in your shoulders and neck…Is it easier to notice sensations in your shoulders…or in your neck?…It doesn't really matter, just so you are aware of your own experience as it occurs.

Now bring your awareness to your face…exploring and discovering the sensations that are occurring in your face…And now your awareness sinks inside your head.

Spread your attention throughout your entire body…becoming more and more aware of your whole inner body…your inner being and all the feelings and sensations that come and go as you become more and more aware of the presence of your inner body…Experience it rather than think about it.

Now, without changing it in any way, turn your attention to your breath…and notice your breathing just as it is…Leave it alone…Don't try and change it in any way…More and more, simply be mindful of the incoming and outgoing breath. When your mind starts to think, let go of the thoughts and return your awareness to your breath.

Shift your awareness to your mood…What emotions and feelings do you notice? Make room for all the feelings and sensations as they come and go…Once again, there's no need to name them…Instead, notice how the feelings land for you physically…Where are they felt in your body?…Are they most noticeable in your gut…or in your heart area…or possibly around your face?…Where else do you feel them? Notice what happens to your emotions when you experience them physically.

Again, take another big breath in…and sigh it out.

Guide your awareness to wherever you would like…as long as it is happening in this present moment…It could be your physical presence…your emotions…your breath…even the sounds in the room…just so it's something that's happening right now.

Pause.

Become aware of the part of you that notices your body, mind and emotions and rest your awareness there.

Pause

Bring your attention back to the room you are in … Sense it or see it around you. Notice if anything has shifted inside during this time.

Whenever you feel like it … stretch your body … and when you feel ready, open your eyes and look around.

Squeeze Stress Away

Guided Relaxation

Time: 15 minutes

Summary: Progressive muscular relaxation to relax your body, mind, and emotions.

This is a time for you to relax and take it easy for a while...doing so will restore your energy to a level that's just right for you...Take a moment to get into a comfortable position either sitting or lying down. Shift around until you are feeling comfortable with where you are.

Let your eyes softly close and take a rest...Turn your attention away from the outside world and notice how you feel right now...Notice any places that feel tired or tense...becoming aware of the physical sensations that you're feeling...There's no need to even name them or judge them...simply notice how your body is feeling right now.

Take in a full, deep breath through your nose...and now, sigh it out through an open mouth.

Pause.

Breathe in again, letting the air go all the way in...and sigh it out completely...Let all of the tiredness, tension, and negativity be released with your breath.

Now, let your breath become slow and easy...Slowly, breathe all the way in...and all the way out...and each time you breathe out, feel yourself releasing any tension you may have...Tension may be in the form of physical tightness...mental confusion...or emotional stress...Each time you exhale...just let it clear away...Notice how the relaxation increases each time you exhale.

For now, allow yourself to forget about the past and let go of the future so you can stay focused upon each and every present moment...softly focusing on your breath.

Next, you're going to tense and then release your muscles...to let go of more and more tension...and to replace it with a sense of relief.

Bring your attention to your right leg...and from your toes to your hips, start tensing the muscles...feeling the squeeze, squeeze it right on in...and now, all at once, release and let go...releasing all the muscular tightness and tension...feel the relief and relaxation in your leg.

Shift your attention to your left leg...Squeeze it and feel it from your toes to your thigh. Know it, hold it, feel the energy...and relax, letting go.

And now, let your legs rest. Become fully aware of the different way tension and relaxation feels to you.

Let your feet relax completely...allow your ankles to release...Now allow your calves...thighs...and hips to let go of tension...more and more. Let your legs feel totally supported now...Notice if they are warm and comfortable...perhaps feeling heavier and heavier...and now, resolve to let your legs stay still for a while.

Draw your attention to your hips and buttocks. Squeeze the muscles, feeling the energy...and melt, letting it all go, feeling the relief...and let the relief spread.

Bring your awareness to your navel. Pull your muscles in and feel the press...now relax...allowing the knots to untie. And let it happen.

This time, push your navel area outward...and feel the abdominal wall stretch...Now let go. You are feeling more and more calm and relaxed. Notice the general well-being that comes with relaxing around your navel.

Bring your awareness around your heart and lungs...Take a full breath in and hold it briefly, feel it for a moment...and all at once let it all go.

Now breathe down into the space deep inside...softly and smoothly...and each time you breathe out, notice how your chest and abdomen relax more and more...letting the tension dissolve, as your relaxation grows deeper. And you allow it to happen.

Shift your attention to your right arm. Squeeze your hand into a tight ball...feel it...Add a squeeze for your arm...and all the way up to your shoulder...Now spread your fingers out...and relax, releasing entirely.

Shift your attention to your left arm. Squeeze your hand into a tight ball...feel it...Add on a squeeze for your arm...and all the way up to your shoulder...Now spread your fingers out...and relax, releasing entirely. Being aware of the relaxation spreading through and through.

Your fingers relax...your hands soften...Feel your arms and shoulders letting go into the comfort and safety of relaxation. More and more ... feel the relaxation and enjoy it ... feeling comfortable and at ease and resolving to let your arms stay still.

Focus your attention on your face. To relax your mouth and jaw, open your mouth and move your jaw up and down and all around ... and now relax, letting your teeth part slightly ... Press your tongue against the roof of your mouth or back of your teeth ... feel it ... and now let go ... softening inside, resting your tongue softly in your mouth ... Softening the corners of your lips ... letting go completely into the comfort of relaxation.

This time, squeeze your nose and cheeks ... and now release and let go.

Even though your eyes are already closed, squeeze your eyes and forehead ... and now relax ... feeling your forehead smoothing out ... and your eyes resting completely ... allowing the corners of your eyes to rest.

Feel yourself become more and more relaxed and rested.

Notice how soft your breathing has become ... just let it be ... and each time you breathe, notice how much more you can relax, deeper and deeper. And the more you relax, the more room there will be for your energy to return to you.

Longer pause.

Now it's time to deepen your breath, and each time you breathe in, feel your energy returning ... feeling more and more refreshed with each and every breath.

Pause.

Whenever you're ready, you can begin to stretch and move, feeling refreshed and renewed.

Recorded on *Wholesome Energizers* CD by Julie Lusk with music by Tom Laskey. Available from Whole Person Associates at 800-247-6789 or on the Web at wholeperson.com.

Breathe, Relax, Feel, Watch, and Allow Meditation

Guided Relaxation and Meditation

Contributed by Sudhir Jonathan Foust

Time: 15 to 20 minutes

Summary: Consciously or unconsciously, we constantly seek a dynamic balance of free-flowing energy and spacious awareness. The following meditation allows you to be present to the process of life unfolding moment by moment and will guide you into a dynamic state of relaxed awareness.

Take a few long full deep breaths... slow, deep and full. Notice how much you can expand your belly and lungs on the inhalation... Notice how much you can soften on the exhalation.

In your own time, let go of all control of your breath. Simply now, observe your breath.

Feel your breath moving in your belly as you breathe... Feel your breath moving through your lungs as you breathe... Feel your breath moving through the sinus cavities in your head as you breathe... Feel your breath moving through your nostrils, noticing perhaps if one nostril is more open than the other.

As you observe your body breathing, notice if your breath is more predominant in one area... perhaps with the rising and falling of your belly... perhaps with the sensation of breath at the rim of your nostrils.

Allow yourself to focus on one particular area of your breath, perhaps your belly or your nostrils... Allow your awareness to rest there... using the sensation of breath as the focal point for your awareness.

When you notice your mind wandering, return again and again to the direct experience of the body breathing in this moment.

As you feel your breath, relax the muscles of your face... Let your face be like the face of a marble statue... Relax your lips and your tongue... Relax your throat and your neck... Relax your shoulders and your arms, elbows and palms... Relax your belly and your lower back... Relax your hips... your knees... your ankles... and the soles of your feet.

Effortless breath... relaxed body.

Observe who you are as a being of sensation ... a being of feeling... feeling the points of contact between your body and that which is supporting you... feeling the vibration of the sounds around you... feeling the texture and the temperature of the air touching your skin.

Feeling all the qualities of your physical body... feeling the qualities of your emotional body... the quality of your heart... the feeling tone of your body.

Breathing, relaxing, feeling.

Invoking a quality of spacious awareness... acknowledging your linear rational mind that serves to compare and judge and seek understanding ... and in your own way, acknowledging that which is beyond your rational mind.

The realm of presence... the realm of who you are with no preferences... observing your capacity to allow the moment to unfold in its own way, its own time.

Let your awareness be like a vast, spacious sky ... feelings ... thoughts... and sensations constantly changing form and shape

As you notice your mind caught up into the past or the future, return again and again to the present moment of the breath, the flow of sensation, the flow of the moment... being present to the process of life unfolding moment by moment.

Where is your breath? ... Where is your mind? ...

Soften your body around the breath. Relax and soften into sensation as the witness, the observer.

Nowhere to go... nothing to do... only to be.

Be present to the moment...

Feel the radiance of effortlessness.

Who are you in the absence of struggle?

Who are you undefended or not distracted?

Radiate out the fullness of who you are.

Let go into effortless being.

When you feel ready, let your breath deepen slightly and open your eyes.

Contributed by Sudhir Jonathan Foust from his *Energy Awareness* CD, which is available from The Relaxation Company by calling 800-788-6670 or through therelaxationcompany.com.

Sudhir Jonathan Foust is the past president of the Kripalu Center for Yoga and Health, the largest yoga center in North America. Sudhir has studied and practiced numerous approaches to meditation from both the Yogic and Buddhist traditions. He is also a senior teacher at Kripalu Center, a mind-body therapist, a teacher trainer, and leader of a variety of seminars and retreats designed to help people cultivate a living relationship to spirit. His CD recordings include, *The Art of Relaxation, A Touch of Grace: Bamboo Flute Meditations,* and *Energy Awareness Meditations,* produced in conjunction with The Relaxation Company and Simon & Schuster.

Warm Hands

Guided Autogenic Relaxation

Contributed by Nancy Loving Tubesing and Donald A Tubesing

Time: 5 to 10 minutes

Summary: Use the power of suggestion to reverse the physical effects of stress. This soothing autogenic routine helps muscles to relax, allowing blood to circulate freely to all parts of the body. It is especially effective for headaches or insomnia.

() () ()

Lean back and relax, as comfortably as possible ... you may want to close your eyes to reduce distractions.

Begin by taking a deep breath ... Inhale, filling your lungs with air all the way down to the belly.

Now exhale slowly with a soft "whooshing" sound ... Take another deep breath ... and imagine as you breathe out that all the tension is leaving your body.

Imagine your hands as warm ... relaxed and warm ... Say to yourself slowly ...

My hands are warm ... relaxed and warm ...

My hands are warm ... relaxed and warm ...

My hands are warm ... relaxed and warm ...

My hands are warm ... relaxed and warm ...

Now visualize your hands in a bucket of warm water ... or comfortably near a roaring fire.

Stay with the image as you slowly say to yourself ... my hands are warm.

Pause.

Make your mental image as vivid as possible as you warm your hands in this comfortable cozy way ... reminding yourself again ...

My hands are warm … relaxed and warm …

Pause.

As you continue to visualize your hands becoming warmer and more relaxed … perhaps you can allow the blood to flow down your arms … and into your hands … allowing them to feel warmer and warmer … more and more relaxed.

Let that feeling of warmth and relaxation spread down your arms and into your hands as you say to yourself …

My hands are warm … relaxed and warm …

Pause.

Now allow that pleasant feeling of warmth to spread throughout your body as you tell yourself … I am calm and relaxed.

Pause.

Continue to enjoy this feeling of warmth and relaxation as you prepare to turn your attention from the inner you to the outer world.

Before you open your eyes … mentally prepare for your return by saying several times to yourself …

When I open my eyes, I will feel relaxed, fresh, and alert.

Pause.

When you are ready … please open your eyes.

Contributed by Nancy Loving Tubesing and Donald A. Tubesing. "Warm Hands" is published in *Relaxation Scripts for Harmony, Tranquility, Serenity* and in *Structured Exercises in Stress Management, Vol. 3.* It is also available on the CD and audiotape *Warm and Heavy.* You may purchase it at wholeperson.com or by calling 800-247-6789.

Complete Relaxation with Yoga Nidra

Guided Relaxation

Nidra is pronounced NEE-drah

Time: 20 to 30 minutes

Summary: Yoga Nidra is the term that means yogic sleep. It refers to the state of complete relaxation in which the body profoundly relaxes, the thinking mind subsides, but awareness remains. When this happens, intuitive knowing and deep peace and joy are awakened.

About 3000 years ago, a map of the body of being was presented in the Taittiriya Upanishad. It outlines five layers, or sheaths of being, called the koshas. These layers include the physical body (anna-maya kosha), the prana energy body (prana-maya kosha), the mental/emotional body (mano-maya-kosha), the intuitive/wisdom body (vijnana-maya kosha) and the spirit or bliss body (ananda-maya kosha).

Understanding and knowing how the koshas work will give you the means to go into a very deep stage of relaxation and expanded awareness. This takes place when a weightless, timeless, peaceful state of being occurs. For this to happen, a process is done in progressive stages designed to systematically relax the physical body, the prana energy body, the mind, emotions, and senses. As each of these layers (koshas) is put to rest, the experience of relaxation changes. It begins with the sensation of bodily heaviness as the muscles are relieved of tension. This is accomplished using progressive muscular relaxation.

In the next stage, the energy body is relaxed through conscious breathing, and an inner stillness is experienced within the heaviness. At this point, the breath becomes very shallow and subtle and is used to calm the thinking mind, soothe the emotions, and still the senses. This is when the feeling of physical heaviness lifts and a lightness of being occurs. Once this happens, intuitive wisdom can be recognized because the thinking mind is at rest. A temporary detachment from worldly affairs and an awareness of being that is beyond the body-mind occurs. A sense of weightlessness is experienced and brings about profound relaxation, absolute stillness, and a sense of joyful well-being

❂ ❂ ❂

This is a time to deeply relax ... it's a special time for self-discovery and restoration on many levels. Deep relaxation is a unique feeling of being deeply relaxed and yet aware, alert and awake.

Arrange any necessary props for maximum comfort ... Stretch out on the floor and close your eyes ... Let your heels be about two feet apart. This will help relax your hips and legs. Feel free to make your own personal adjustments so your legs and hips feel very comfortable ... allow your feet and toes to open out to the sides and rest ... Now, notice your hips ... feel where your hips rest upon the ground ... lift them up slightly and settle them back down ... nice and even ... nice and easy.

Now, notice your shoulders. Feel where your shoulders are placed ... Gently, circle them up, back and down so your shoulder blades can rest comfortably beneath you ... supporting you ... Gently rock your head from side to side a few times ... Now, position your head and neck so they are in alignment with your spine ... Feel free to adjust your clothing and props ... and position every part of your body so that you are very, very comfortable.

Now, bring your awareness to your right leg, from your foot on up to your hip ... Begin to tense the muscles ... just squeeze the muscles ... and feel the squeeze ... and now, all at once, relax, letting all the tension drain away ... Notice the muscles relax ... feeling heavy and relaxed.

Bring your awareness to your left leg, from your foot on up to your hip ... Begin to hug the muscles in to the bones ... feel the squeeze ... and now let go totally ... let go, allowing your leg to relax ... noticing a comfortable heaviness in both of your legs as they relax more and more.

Bring your awareness to your buttocks and squeeze these muscles ... Feel the squeeze ... and now relax, feeling these muscles melt like honey in hot tea ... allowing all the tightness and tension to drain away from around your hips.

Begin squeezing your naval inward and feel the squeeze ... pressing the naval in ... and now relax and soften the naval area ... relaxing and softening, more and more ... This time push your naval outward and feel the abdominal wall stretch ... hold ... and relax ... softening the muscles more and more ... Each time you softly breathe out ... you can relax even more ... letting go of tension.

Bring your awareness to your right arm, becoming aware of your arm from your hand on up to your shoulder ... Tighten your hand into a fist ... and move the tension up your arm to your shoulder ... Now open

your fingers up...and all at once, let go of all the squeezing and tension...feeling the muscles relax...Compare and contrast the sensations
of squeezing and relaxing...and letting go into the heaviness and comfort
of relaxation...comparing and contrasting with your mind's eye.

Shift your awareness over to your left hand and make a tight fist...Feel the
squeeze go into your arm and up to your shoulder...Spread your fingers
out wide...and finally, totally let go...feeling the heaviness and comfort
of relaxation spreading through your shoulders, arms, and hands.

Notice how your mind can be alert, even as your body relaxes more
and more...and notice the heaviness, the feeling of muscular relaxation...sinking into stillness.

Bring your awareness to your jaw...Open your mouth and move your
jaw all around, letting go of tension in your jaw...and now relax and
become still...letting your teeth part slightly...relaxing the corners of
your lips...You can even moisten your lips if you'd like...Now press
your tongue against the roof of your mouth or to the back of your
teeth and let go...relaxing your tongue and resting it softly in your
mouth...Notice the openness and hollowness inside.

Even though your eyes are closed, squeeze your eyes...and your forehead
and feel the squeeze... Now let go...and your forehead smoothes out
like satin.

Feel your body resting deeply...content and comforted by the relaxation.

Just for a moment, barely open your eyes...and let them close...feel the
relief...Can you feel where your eyelids touch?

Pause.

If you would like to relax further now, you can...just become more and
more aware of your breath.

Bring your awareness to your legs...Without moving your legs, take a
conscious breath in...Then breathe out and feel your legs relax, more
and more...and now, bring your awareness to your hips...breathing
mindfully...and being aware of your hips, allowing your conscious
breath to relax your hips even more...letting go with each and every
exhalation...feeling the heaviness of relaxation...and the stillness.

Now bring your awareness to your belly...Take a deep breath in and
breathing out, let go of all tension in and around your belly...Bring
your awareness around your heart and lungs and take a big, full breath
in...all the way...and exhale...Your chest settles into relaxation...yet

your mind is alert and aware of what is happening... breathing and allowing your awareness to rest all around your heart.

Bring your awareness to your arms. Take a breath in, consciously breathing in... breathe out and let your arms rest and relax.

Bring your awareness to your head... Take another big deep breath in and relax your face.

Letting all of the muscles relax... your body relaxes totally... Notice how comfortable and heavy your muscles feel... feeling a blanket of relaxation covering you with quietness and calmness.

Notice what you're experiencing right here and now.

Pause.

If you'd like, feel free to shift around a little or adjust your clothes.

Pause.

Notice how soft and subtle your breath has become... Let it be... allowing your breath to be soft and subtle.

Perhaps you'd like to go further into relaxation... If you would, simply follow your natural, soft breath with your attention and your awareness.

Bring your attention back to your legs and let your breath be like a sweeping motion, sweeping down your legs with your breath, erasing thoughts, memories and feelings... brushing the tension away with your soft and subtle breath... removing thoughts... memories... Old injuries are swept clean with your breath as it flows down your legs.

Perhaps you notice the heaviness being replaced with a lighter feeling... and lighter still.

Bring your awareness around your hips and with your soft subtle breath, sweep tensions away, allowing your breath to release old pain... sweeping it away and allowing relaxation to happen more and more.

And as relaxation deepens, it feels as if you're floating.

If you feel uncomfortable at any time, simply open your eyes for a bit or shift your body around somewhat.

Feel the sweeping and brushing breath in and around the vital organs of your abdomen... softening and lightening... releasing tension and old hurts with your breath... removing any remaining tension with your subtle breath in and around your vital organs... and it lessens and lightens with the soft and subtle breath ... And now this sweeping motion moves around your heart ... and old memories, feelings, and tensions are cleared away with your breath ... fresh and clean.

Your breath naturally begins sweeping down your arms now ... removing thoughts, feelings and memories, and your arms feel light and easy ... as if they're floating.

Feeling quite peaceful, use this technique around your neck and throat ... and as the tensions release, the connection between your head and heart opens and becomes free and clear and easy ... simply brushing with your gentle breath.

And now sweeping and smoothing out around your ears ... softening more and more ... your sense of inner hearing is awakened ... and now your breath brushes all around your eyes ... and your inner eyes open and inner sight clears ... and let the last bit of tension leave through the top of your head.

Observe the lightness ... the softness ... the weightlessness of deep relaxation ... feeling detached from your body ... and mind ... and from worldly cares ... just for now.

Pause one minute.

For a moment now, stretch just a little bit ... perhaps, move a finger just a little bit or open your eyes slightly ... and settle back into the richness of relaxation.

If you like, you can go further and deeper still by looking for a place, sensing a place inside where inner joy resides ... a place to rest in silence and tranquility ... a place to experience connection and completeness ... Your awareness is open and very still.

Pause five minutes.

It's time to make the transition back ... Without having to move in any way, bring your awareness back to the body ... and slowly return your attention to the breath ... and simply follow the breath with your awareness.

Bring your awareness to the heart center and to your breathing ... becoming more and more aware of your body.

Bring your awareness to the top of your head and feel your head and face awaken ... Your sense of seeing ... and hearing awakens as you become more and more aware, listening to the sounds in the room.

And now your attention flows to your neck...If you'd like, slowly roll your neck and head from side to side...Feel the movement...and let yourself become still again.

Your awareness flows down the back of your body through your spine...and through the front of your body...and through your heart...your lungs...and your vital organs...Now your awareness flows into your arms...and hands...wiggle your fingers around just a bit and stretch your arms...and now wiggle your toes around and stretch your legs.

Bring your awareness back to your eyes...Even though they are still closed, you notice more and more light coming through...and now begin to stretch more and more...moving and waking up your body and mind.

When you're ready, roll over onto your side and curl up.

Long pause.

To raise yourself to a sitting position, press your hands and arms down to lift yourself up.

Allow your eyes to close again and relish the stillness...

Open your eyes just a sliver...notice more light...then close them again and rest...Slowly blink your eyes open and closed to blend the inner world with the outer world...When your eyes are completely open, you'll be awake and alert, yet relaxed.

Authors Note: Many thanks to Nischala Joy Devi who guided me through my first experience of this technique and helped me recognize the different stages of relaxation through the understanding and use of the koshas.

Affirmations for Energy, Strength, and Inner Vitality

Guided Relaxation and Affirmations

Time: 15 minutes

Summary: Affirmations are coupled with the breath to increase your energy, inner strength, and vitality. Repeat the following statements to yourself, silently or out loud, and in time with the rhythm of your natural breath. While each phrase appears only twice, be sure to take enough time to connect with each one, particularly the ones that hold the most meaning to you.

Variations: Feel free to modify the following verses until you find the version that feels right for you. For example, instead of "Breathing in, plant courage … breathing out, feel courage grow," use "Breathing in, may I plant courage … breathing out, may I feel courage grow." Another idea is to say, "Breathing in, I plant courage … breathing out, I feel courage grow." You may also add more verses or simply practice the ones that are most meaningful to you.

It's time to use affirmations and the power of your mind and intention to increase your energy, inner strength and vitality. Allow the following statements to echo in your mind letting the affirmations flow through you, refreshing and renewing you … repeating them to yourself … allowing them to soak deep inside … If an affirmation doesn't seem to fit you, don't worry, just breathe softly and wait for the next one … or change it to suit yourself, just so it's still positive … or simply pretend that it's true.

Combining affirmations with the power of your breath is especially potent. All you have to do is repeat the statements to yourself in time with the rhythm of your natural breath.

You may either lie on your back or sit in a meditative posture … Stretch comfortably and move around until you feel settled and comfortable.

Take a big breath in … and sigh it out.

Be still for a few moments and feel your body softening into the comfort of relaxation ... Breathe in a way that is slow and smooth ... evening out your inhalations and exhalations. Doing so, in and of itself, will release tension and replace it with waves of energy.

And now, as you breathe slowly and smoothly, allow your awareness to expand and make room for your imagination and for positive affirmations to reclaim your inner strength and energy.

It may help if you imagine that you are like a garden as you plant positive, affirming qualities within yourself to help them grow and develop.

Breathing in, feel your lungs expand ... breathing out, let go.
Breathing in, feel your lungs expand ... breathing out, let go.

Breathing in, plant strength ... breathing out, feel strength grow.
Breathing in, plant strength ... breathing out, feel strength grow.

Breathing in, plant courage ... breathing out, feel courage grow.
Breathing in, plant courage ... breathing out, feel courage grow.

Breathing in, plant hope ... breathing out, feel hope grow.
Breathing in, plant hope ... breathing out, feel hope grow.

Breathing in, plant steadiness ... breathing out, feel steadiness grow.
Breathing in, plant steadiness ... breathing out, feel steadiness grow.

Breathing in, plant vibrant health ... breathing out, feel vibrant health grow.
Breathing in, plant vibrant health ... breathing out, feel vibrant health grow.

Breathing in, plant acceptance ... breathing out, feel acceptance grow.
Breathing in, plant acceptance ... breathing out, feel acceptance grow.

Breathing in, plant forgiveness ... breathing out, feel forgiveness grow.
Breathing in, plant forgiveness ... breathing out, feel forgiveness grow.

Breathing in, plant love ... breathing out, feel love grow.
Breathing in, plant love ... breathing out, feel love grow.

Breathing in, plant contentment ... breathing out, feel contentment grow.
Breathing in, plant contentment ... breathing out, feel contentment grow.

Breathing in, plant clarity ... breathing out, feel clarity grow.
Breathing in, plant clarity ... breathing out, feel clarity grow.

Breathing in, plant playfulness ... breathing out, feel playfulness grow.
Breathing in, plant playfulness ... breathing out, feel playfulness grow.

Breathing in, plant patience ... breathing out, feel patience grow.
Breathing in, plant patience ... breathing out, feel patience grow.

Breathing in, plant gratitude ... breathing out, feel gratitude grow.
Breathing in, plant gratitude ... breathing out, feel gratitude grow.

Breathing in, plant confidence ... breathing out, feel confidence grow.
Breathing in, plant confidence ... breathing out, feel confidence grow.

Breathing in, plant trust ... breathing out, feel trust grow.
Breathing in, plant trust ... breathing out, feel trust grow.

Breathing in, plant wholeness ... breathing out, feel wholeness grow.
Breathing in, plant wholeness ... breathing out, feel wholeness grow.

Continue on your own, planting those qualities that are especially meaningful to you and when you're ready, stretch, open your eyes, and enjoy feeling refreshed and restored. Remember these qualities throughout the day and watch them grow.

Breathing Practices
Your Portable Paradise

*The breathing practices stabilize and balance
the flow of breath and increase life energy.*
Yoga Sutra 2.49

Yogis from ancient times were as interested in increasing life energy as we are today. Breathing practices and breath patterns will give us that energy and serve as a bridge reconnecting the life force inherent in our mind and body.

Breathwork plays an important role in the practice of relaxation, imagery, and meditation and contributes significantly to mind-body health.

Physically, focused breathing oxygenates all the cells, tissues and organs, slows the heart rate, improves digestion and elimination, nourishes the brain, and regulates the nervous system.

Mentally, focused breathing encourages concentration by bringing attention back to the breath each time the mind wanders. Memory is improved because the brain gets the nourishment it needs from proper oxygenization, resulting in clear thinking and better mental functioning.

Emotionally, focused breathing eases uncomfortable feelings and brings feelings of evenness and equanimity through the acknowledgement, observation, acceptance, and release of emotions.

Spiritually, focused breathing creates spaciousness and opens the doorway to inner stillness, insight, and wisdom.

The following breathing practices come from the yoga tradition. They are as valid today as they were thousands of years ago.

The Complete Breath: Dirgha Breathing (5 minutes or longer)

Ocean Breath: Ujjayi Breath (5 minutes or longer)

Alternate Nostril Breathing: Nadi Shodhana (2 minutes or longer)

Breath of Fire: Kapalabhati (5 minutes or longer)

The Complete Breath
Dirgha Breathing

Breathing Practice

Dirgha is pronounced DEAR-gah

Time: 5 minutes or longer

Summary: This breathing technique is done with long, slow, deep breaths while focusing on the lower, mid, and upper portions of your chest. This allows for the fullest breathing possible and will improve respiration, circulation, and even digestion. The complete breath will soothe your frazzled nerves, clear your mind, and replenish your life force.

> *Controlling the volume, duration and frequency of the inhalation, the*
> *exhalation, and the pauses between each breath enhances prana,*
> *the energy that supports and sustains the life force.*
> *Breathing becomes slow and refined.*
>
> Yoga Sutra 2.50

Come into a comfortable seated position with your spine erect or lie on your back. First, practice this technique while lying on your back because it is easy to learn in that position. Next, practice it while sitting upright. Be sure to breathe in this manner during other activities. Not only will you reap the benefits of better respiration, you'll be practicing mindfulness.

Breathing through your nose is optimal because it prepares the air for the lungs by filtering, warming, and moistening it. However if your nose is blocked, breathe through your mouth to the degree that it is necessary.

Begin with a full exhalation to expel stale air and carbon dioxide and make room for a full, deep inhalation. A slow and complete exhalation also activates the relaxation response. When exhaling, allow your breath to flow out of your lungs in the most relaxed and natural way. Just before the end of the exhalation, contract your abdominal muscles slightly to squeeze residual air out of your lungs and to empty them completely.

Take time to fill your torso completely while inhaling. To do so, first relax and release your abdomen. Feel the muscles in your abdominal region expand as the air comes in. Continue inhaling, while expanding your lower chest and ribs and then your upper chest until your collarbones rise slightly. Feel each section expanding naturally in a wave-like motion from the bottom to the top. If it is hard for you to feel this, watch it happen.

Continue breathing deeply while keeping the rest of your body relaxed. Let your breathing be smooth, even, and uninterrupted. After you are accustomed to breathing fully and completely, practice regulating your breath so your inhalation and your exhalation are equal in duration. In other words, breathe in to the count of four and breathe out to the count of four (om one, om two, etc.). This is called a 1: 1 ratio. When this is easy and natural for you, start lengthening the exhalation to activate the relaxation response. This is done by breathing in to the count of four and breathing out to the count of eight. This is called a 1:2 ratio. Remember not to strain or struggle.

Practice the complete breath frequently throughout the day. Doing so will improve your lung capacity and will reward you with the gifts of mindfulness.

If you notice feeling lightheaded or dizzy, lessen your effort until these sensations pass, then try again. Your system is probably not used to this new ratio of oxygen to carbon dioxide yet. If you feel the need to gasp for air while breathing, you are trying too hard. Let the air stream flow easily and fully.

Please note that it is important that your abdominal muscles naturally expand and inflate while inhaling. This is due to the action of the respiratory diaphragm as it raises and lowers during breathing; therefore, there is no need to purposefully or mechanically use your abdominal muscles to inhale. Just watch a baby breathe and you will see this happen. This is the correct way to breathe, and it will optimize all the benefits of respiration.

You are a reverse breather if you feel your belly pull in while inhaling. Make every effort to correct this faulty breathing pattern. Allowing your belly to expand rather than contract when inhaling can change this pattern. Reverse breathers are prone to chronic tension in the upper body, especially around the jaw, neck, upper back and shoulders. It can contribute to mental confusion, heartburn, indigestion, bloating, and gas.

Chest breathing, also called paradoxical breathing, occurs when you primarily breathe with your upper chest, restricting the movement of the breath in the abdomen. This is a very inefficient way to breathe because it does not allow for full oxygenization. Chest breathing triggers the flight or fight response, and this results in feeling on edge or anxious most of the time. Chest breathers are more prone to hypertension and heart disease. It also restricts movement and circulation in the vital organs in the abdomen and leads to chronic tension in the back, shoulders, and neck.

The solution for reverse and chest breathing is to practice breathing deeply and fully while consciously allowing your belly to move out on the inhalation and in on the exhalation. It will help if you lie on your back, place your hands on your belly, and practice natural abdominal breathing as described above.

Ocean Breath
Ujjayi Breath

Breathing Practice

Ujjayi is pronounced oo-JAH-yee or sometimes "ooo" as in cool and "ji" as in hi.

Time: 5 minutes or longer

Summary: The Ujjayi Breath, also called the Ocean Sounding Breath, is a yogic breathing practice that builds on the benefits of Dirgha Breathing, the complete breath. Meditative and calming, it creates concentration while it develops stamina and endurance. This breath helps relieve sinus problems and can diminish headache pain.

The Ujjayi is performed by taking long, slow, and deep breaths (the complete dirgha pranayama) while creating a special sound in the back of the throat that sounds like ocean waves.

Although you will breathe in and out through your nose when doing Ujjayi, it is easier to learn first by breathing through an open mouth while whispering the sound of "home" or "Om." Doing so will allow you to experience the open feeling in your throat that is used in Ujjayi breathing. When practicing, notice how your lips are slightly open when whispering the "ho" or "o" sound. Also notice the hollow, open feeling in your throat. Maintain the open sensation in your throat as the sound changes into "mmm." Listen to the sound at the back of your throat as you continue breathing out. Repeat several times, drawing out the "mmm" sound more and more each time. This is the Ujjayi sound, a unique, audible Darth Vader-type sound. This same sound and feeling in your throat is used for the inhalation as well.

Next, close your mouth and continue breathing in and out through your nostrils while maintaining that feeling and sound in your throat. When done correctly, there is a slight constriction in the glottis (the opening between the vocal chords) during inhalation and exhalation. Ujjayi breathing can be practiced any time, anywhere.

Either come into a comfortable seated position with your spine erect or lie on your back.

Begin by taking long, slow and deep breaths through your nostrils.

Allow your breath to be gentle and relaxed as you slightly contract the back of your throat creating a steady ocean sound as you breathe in and out. The sound need not be forced, but it should be loud enough so that if someone came close to you they would hear it.

Gradually, lengthen the inhalation and the exhalation as much as possible without creating tension anywhere in your body, and allow the sound of the breath to be continuous and smooth. Keep the pitch and intensity of the breath consistent and even throughout. As you begin, practice breathing so both your inhalation and exhalation are equal in length and duration; then lengthen the exhalation as done in the Complete Dirgha Breath.

Continue practicing, allowing your inhalations and exhalations to follow a circular flow that is continuous and almost seamless, leaving as little space between the incoming and outgoing breath as possible. Remember to relax into your breathing; there is no reason to rush.

After your Ujjayi breath becomes smooth and seamless, practice another breathing pattern by holding your breath for a few seconds at the end of the inhalation and/or at the end of the exhalation. This tends to produce more focus. However, never hold your breath if you have high blood pressure.

Alternate Nostril Breathing
Nadi Shodhana

Breathing Practice: Three patterns and five breathing ratios

Nadi Shodhana is pronounced NAH-dee SHOW-dah-nah.

Time: 2 minutes of daily practice. Increase gradually to 10 minutes or longer.

Summary: Alternate nostril breathing creates a sense of physical, mental and emotional well-being. This yogic breath is done by alternating nostrils while breathing. Doing so balances right and left-brain integration, promoting mental clarity and whole brain functioning. It can relieve sinus problems and most headaches. It calms emotions and fosters feelings of deep inner contentment and balance. Due to its calming effect, it is ideal as preparation for deep relaxation or meditation.

Nadi Shodhana is well known for balancing the nadis (pronounced NAH-deez), the nonphysical nerve channels within the body. Yogis say that prana, the life force, is distributed through the nadis. While there are considered to be over 72,000 nadis that travel throughout the body, there are three primary ones that run along the spine.

The ida (pronounced EE-dah) is to the left of the spine and corresponds to the right side of the brain. It is activated by the exhalation and is associated with receptiveness, intuition, and passivity.

The pingala (pronounced pin-GAH-lah) is to the right of the spine and corresponds to the left side of the brain. It is activated by the inhalation and is associated with activity, logic, and objectivity.

The sushumna (pronounced sue-SHOOM-nah) is the central channel within the spine, located in the hollow at the back of the spine where the spinal cord extends from the sacrum to the skull, and is activated by the gap between breaths. It is linked with wisdom and the balancing of our active and receptive nature. Of particular interest, the ida and pingala intertwine around the first four chakras, and the practice of Nadi Shodhana will balance and lift this powerful energy all the way to the crown chakra.

The first step to the practice is to learn the proper hand position to aid in the alternation of the breath. Two hand positions are offered, and both are effective. Try them both to find out which feels easier for you. Take a few minutes to get used to switching between nostrils with the hand positions before adding the breathing patterns.

To try the first position, Vishnu Mudra, bend the index and middle finger of your right hand toward your palm. This will leave your thumb, ring and pinky fingers upright. Next, gently close your right nostril with your thumb; then release your thumb and close your left nostril with the ring finger of your right hand. Switch back and forth until it feels smooth.

Nasagra Mudra is another hand position that can be used. Begin by making the peace sign with your right hand. Next, bring your pointer and middle fingers together and then release your thumb. Place the pads of your index and middle fingers in the center of your forehead or between your eyebrows and then use your thumb and the knuckle of your ring finger to alternately close and release your nostrils.

Three breathing patterns are offered. Take your time and practice each pattern daily for a week or more. You will notice that each pattern has a slightly different effect. All three are based on deep, even breathing that is symmetrical and balanced with the exhalation and inhalation equal in depth and duration. Always start with an exhalation. Dirgha or Dirgha/Ujjayi breathing is recommended. The rhythm of the inhalation to the exhalation is usually uneven at first, but it will smooth out with practice so that the inhalation and exhalation become equal in length. When this is easy for you, begin slowing the exhalation so that it becomes longer than the inhalation until eventually the exhalation is twice as long as your inhalation. Additional ratios are offered below. Maintain alertness to your breath instead of breathing mechanically.

Pattern One: Nadi Shodhana

Come into a comfortable seated position with your spine erect. While either hand position can be used, the Vishnu Mudra is used to describe the pattern for the sake of clarity. The first pattern alternates nostrils after each inhalation. No counting is required.

Exhale / inhale / change nostril. Exhale / inhale / change nostril. Repeat.

Here's how:

Come into a comfortable seated position with your spine erect.

Form your fingers of your right hand into Vishnu Mudra by curling your index and middle fingers into your palm and place your thumb against your right nostril.

Gently exhale and inhale through your left nostril.

Close the left nostril with the ring finger.

Release the thumb. Gently exhale and inhale through the right nostril.

This is one round.

Repeat, alternating nostrils after each inhalation. Begin practicing for two minutes and gradually, very gradually, increase to ten minutes.

Pattern Two:
Come into a comfortable seated position with your spine erect. Either hand position can be used. Begin practicing for two minutes and gradually, very gradually, increase to ten minutes.

This pattern is done by exhaling and inhaling through one nostril three times followed by changing sides to repeat the pattern through the other nostril. This pattern requires counting.

Left nostril: out / in / out / in / out / in / change nostrils.

Right nostril: out / in / out / in / out / in / change nostrils.

Repeat the sequence.

Pattern Three:
Come into a comfortable seated position with your spine erect. Either hand position can be used. Begin practicing for two minutes and gradually, very gradually, increase to ten minutes.

In this pattern the nostrils are alternated between each inhalation and exhalation for three times per nostril. This pattern requires counting.

Out left / in right / out left / in right / out left / in right / change.

Out right / in left / out right / in left / out right / in left / change.

Out left / in right / out left / in right / out left / in right / change.

Out right / in left / out right / in left / out right / in left / change.

Repeat the sequence.

Breathing Ratio Variations: Take your time with these ratios and never rush. Do not force or strain. Do not use breath retention if you have hypertension or other cardiac conditions.

The examples given are to the count of 4. This can be adjusted to 3, 5, or 6 depending upon your comfort level. Count by silently saying Om 1, Om 2, Om 3, Om 4, etc.

Ratio of 1:1 — Develop breath control so that the inhalation and the exhalation are exactly the same length of time. Inhale for the count of 4. Exhale for 4. Do not proceed until perfected.

Ratio of 1:2 — Double the length of the exhalation. Inhale for the count of 4. Exhale for 8. Do not proceed until perfected.

Ratio of 1:2:2 — Addition of breath retention. Inhale to the count of 4. Hold the breath for 8. Exhale for 8. Do not proceed until perfected.

Ratio of 1:4:2 — Inhale to the count of 4. Hold 16. Exhale 8. Do not proceed until perfected.

Ratio of 1:4:2:3 — Inhale 4. Hold 16. Exhale 8. Hold the exhalation 12. Do not struggle.

Breath of Fire
Kapalabhati

Breathing Practice

Kapalabhati is pronounced KAH-pah-lah-BAH-tee.

Time: 5 minutes or longer

Summary: The Breath of Fire is a powerful breathing technique that emphasizes a pattern of quick exhalations followed by passive inhalations. It cleans and purifies the respiratory system, invigorates the vital organs of digestion, and strengthens the nervous system. Due to the swift and sharp exhalations, a shift in pressure occurs in the cerebral spinal fluid. This causes a massaging effect on the brain, enlivening every cell, and creating an "aura" of light and vitality around the skull. According to yogis, it has a positive influence on both the third and sixth chakras.

Practice three rounds daily. The breath of fire should be practiced on an empty stomach and is not to be practiced if you are pregnant, menstruating or have high blood pressure, recent abdominal surgery, heart disease, severe lung disease, hiatal hernia, or glaucoma. Be cautious if you have digestive or respiratory problems.

Come into a comfortable seated position with your spine erect. Take a few deep, relaxing breaths.

Exhale quickly and completely through the nostrils by contracting (snapping) the abdominal muscles toward the spine. Follow this with a passive inhalation. Repeat this several times slowly. The secret is in the rapid pumping of air out from the lower lobes of the lungs, followed by a passive inhalation that occurs naturally and automatically. The exhalation is active, and the inhalation is passive. To learn the proper amount of effort needed for each exhalation, pretend you are blowing a candle out. As you practice blowing out through your mouth, notice how your abdomen contracts and how your breath is short and quickly releases. In the breath of fire however, your nose is used instead of your mouth.

In the beginning, practice the breath of fire by placing your hands over your naval center. As you exhale, notice how your abdomen quickly moves in toward your spine; as you inhale it will relax as your diaphragm expands with the incoming breath. Keep your shoulders stationary and relaxed and your chest passive.

Once you feel comfortable with coordinating the rapid exhalation, the movement of the abdomen, and the passive inhalation, gradually pick up the pace until you find your own preferred rhythm. Start with ten to fifteen expulsions at first, followed by breathing fully and deeply for three to five complete dirgha breaths. Practice two more sets of ten to fifteen repetitions for a total of three rounds. If you feel dizzy, out of breath, or uncomfortable in any other way, immediately stop and breathe normally until you feel stable again. Progressively increase the number of repetitions per round until you can comfortably do fifty expulsions. There is no need to rush the process. Expect to take several months of daily practice to build up to three rounds of fifty.

Further refinements can be made after you are comfortable with the breath of fire. When you feel at ease with the mechanics of the breath, focus your attention on the middle of your forehead just above your eyebrows, also called the third eye or sixth chakra.

As a further refinement, add a brief period of breath retention between the rounds. To do this, exhale completely on the final exhalation of each round and then pause briefly before inhaling. When you need to, inhale until your lungs are approximately three-fourths full and again pause briefly. Exhale when ready and allow your breath to return to a natural rate.

Guided Breathing Meditations

Breathing exercises stabilize and balance the flow of breath
and increase life energy. The life energy is increased by regulation
of the out-breath, the in-breath, and suspension of the breath.
Breaths are regulated by the volume, length, and frequency of the breath.
Breathing becomes slow and refined.

Yoga Sutra 2.49- 2.50

Enjoy these guided meditations that focus on the breath. They are stabilizing, balancing, and will awaken life energy.

Wholesome Breathing (10 minutes)
Resting in the Gap (10 to 15 minutes)
Energy Breathing (10 to 15 minutes)

Wholesome Breathing

Guided Breathing

Time: 10 minutes

Summary: Full, deep breathing is practiced for relaxation and comfort.

Breathing fully and evenly is a remarkable way to calm yourself, help you focus, and give you comfort and relaxation.

Give yourself a short break to become more aware of your breathing and to bring yourself inner peace ... Begin by taking a big breath in and then sigh it out.

You may either let your eyes softly close and rest or allow them to stay barely open ... If your legs or arms are crossed, uncross them ... and let your whole body settle down, feeling the support of whatever you're resting on ... Move and shift around until you're really comfortable ... Go ahead ... it's fine to let go and settle down ... Take a moment ... tune into your senses here and now ... listening to the sounds around you ... noticing any thoughts or feelings that are now present ... and allowing yourself to let go of your cares and concerns, just for now.

This is a time to renew yourself through the soothing motion of your breath ... All you have to do is bring your awareness to your natural breath ... Notice it's depth ... its pace ... and its rhythm ... simply being aware of your incoming and outgoing breath ... When your mind begins to wander, bring your attention back to your breathing ... breathing through your nose, softly, in and out.

At your own pace, let your incoming breath flow more deeply into your lungs ... and exhale completely and fully ... breathing in and out, slowly and smoothly ... There's no need to rush or hurry ... it will do you good to slow down ... resting in the comfort and steadiness of your breath.

When your mind wanders, gently bring your attention back to your breath.

It's time to become even more aware of your breath ... If you wish, you may place your hand over your navel to help your awareness ... As you're breathing, deeply and slowly, notice how your belly rises up with each inhalation and how it lowers with each exhalation…breathing slowly in…slowly out…feeling the movement of your breath in your body…Breathing in nourishes your cells…breathing out helps you clear out and let go…Your vital organs are receiving a healthy massage from your breath as your belly rises and falls like the tides.

Continue breathing deeply into your belly and bring your attention to your ribs and the sides of your body…As you breathe in slowly permit yourself to feel how your ribs and sides inflate upon inhalation and deflate upon exhalation…breathing in healing oxygen to nourish your entire system…breathing out stale air…nourishing and cleansing as you breathe.

When your mind wanders, gently bring your attention back to your breath.

While your breathing continues…slowly, smoothly, and deeply, draw your attention to the area surrounding your heart…above it, below it…in front and behind it…and now right into its very center…breathing long, easy, and relaxing breaths…Each time you slowly exhale, your heartbeat restores to a healthy pace…and it feels comforting and soothing to be breathing softly, evenly, and fully.

If you'd like to relax further, allow your in breath and out breath to be about equal in length and duration…nice and even…in and out…simply slipping into the easy pace and steadiness of your breath…When your mind wanders, gently bring your attention back to your breath…feeling the air as it easily glides in and out…treasuring your sense of relaxation…Cherishing the feeling of calmness it creates.

Begin stretching and moving around whenever you feel like it…and open your eyes…feeling awake and alert as if you've had a sound night's sleep, and now fully prepared to go on with what comes next.

Recorded on *Wholesome Relaxation* CD by Julie Lusk with music by Tom Laskey. Available from Whole Person Associates at 800-247-6789 or on the Web at wholeperson.com.

Resting in the Gap

Guided Breathing

Time: 15 to 20 minutes or longer

Summary: This relaxing breath brings about an inner stillness, first by focusing on your breath, and then by practicing a three-part exhalation, followed by cultivating awareness of the gap between the exhalation and the inhalation. This gap is known as the midpoint or Madhya in Sanskrit (pronounced mud-yha). It serves as a doorway to the expansion of consciousness and the inner space where the connection to the whole can be experienced.

The intellect is unveiled and illuminated when the breathing practices take us beyond customary perceptions of the internal and external. As sense awareness subsides, the mind is prepared for stillness.
                                                      Yoga Sutra 2.52-2.55

Either sit upright for meditation or lie down on a firm surface. Give yourself the time and permission you need to feel steady and comfortable. Close your eyes or keep them barely open.

Bring your attention to your breath ... and feel the air as it moves in and as it moves back out ... Simply follow the movement of your breath.

Allow your awareness to rest in your heart ... Gradually, allow your breathing to slow down and become longer ... Spend a little more time than usual breathing out, and then breathe in fully ... Continue to give more time to exhaling than to inhaling.

Pause.

When your mind starts wandering, simply bring your attention back to your breathing.

Pause.

Become aware of the pause at the end of your exhalation and before the next inhalation ... it's a tiny space of stillness ... Simply begin to become aware of this little space without trying to change it or lengthen it.

Pause.

To increase your awareness and create a peaceful and quiet feeling inside, you can begin to exhale in three parts.

Here's how. Breathe out one-third of the way, pause briefly, breathe out another third of the way, pause briefly, and then breathe out the remainder of the breath. Then, breathe in slowly and smoothly.

Let's repeat. Breathe out one-third of the way, pause briefly, breathe out another third of the way, pause briefly, and then breathe out the remainder of the breath. Then, breathe in slowly and smoothly. Breathe at a pace that is comfortable for you, without feeling as if you have to force or rush your breath in any way.

Pause for several minutes. Every so often, offer a reminder to bring the mind back to the heart of the breath as well as a reminder of the technique.

Become more and more aware of the pauses in the exhalation … notice the quiet quality that comes within the pauses.

Pause.

Now let go of the three-part pause in the exhalation and breathe out in one smooth exhalation … followed by an inhalation … Continue however, to be aware of the pause at the end of the exhalation and before the inhalation … Take your time to notice this pause … notice what it's like to rest quietly within this pause, calmly waiting for the inhalation to return on its own … followed by another exhalation … and pausing in the gap before the next inhalation. Take your time in the emptiness between the exhalation and the inhalation.

Pause.

When you are ready, begin bringing your attention back to your surroundings. Stretch and open your eyes.

Author's Note: "Resting in the Gap" was inspired by Donna Farhi and her book, *The Breathing Book: Good Health and Vitality Through Essential Breathwork.* New York, Henry Holt and Company, LLC. 1996. The book is wonderful, and so is she.

Energy Breathing

Guided Breathing

Summary: Energy Breathing will center your mind and expand your awareness by focusing your attention on the breath as it rises and falls within the core of your body.

Time: 10 to 15 minutes

Either sit upright for meditation or lie down. Give yourself the time and permission you need to feel steady and comfortable. Close your eyes or keep them barely open.

Bring your awareness to your breath, the easy flow of your breath as it moves in and back out... Become aware of its natural qualities, right now. Begin by letting your breath just be... without trying to change it... without judging it... Let it be... let it be breath.

Become aware of where you notice your breath the most. Perhaps it's at the tip of your nostrils... perhaps you feel it within your body... Center your attention at that place and observe your breath... just as it is. When your mind begins to wander, simply bring your awareness back to your breath.

Pause.

Take another moment or two to settle in more. Feel free to adjust your clothing or reposition your body so you feel as steady and comfortable as you possibly can right now.

While focusing more and more on your breath, place your hands over your navel... Feel the touch of your hands on your body... Experience the exchange of temperature and the connection where your hands meet your body.

When your mind begins to think, come back to the sensation of your hands, resting upon your body, and feel how your hands lift and lower to the rhythm of your breath... Notice the breath moving in your own body... being aware of your breath... and letting go of thoughts... and when thoughts come up, drop them into the stream of your breath so they can be carried away.

Continue drawing your awareness to your navel. When you breathe out, feel your hands sink and lower, and when you breathe in, feel your hands lifted by your belly, breathing smoothly and deeply so your belly gently lifts and lowers with your breath … not because you're muscling and pressing your muscles, but from the action of your breath.

And now bring your hands up until they circle your rib cage. Continue breathing so your ribs expand as you breathe in and compress when you breathe out .… Feel the intercostal muscles open and close. The intercostal muscles are the ones between the ribs and they work like an accordion … Feel your ribs expand and separate as the air comes in and compress as the air leaves.

Now place your hands over your heart and feel where your hands touch your body and notice your breath … Notice how your body moves with your breath as you continue breathing smoothly and evenly.

It's time now to breathe more fully and to unite your awareness and your breath. Leave one hand over your heart and place the other hand over your navel … Inhaling, feel your navel lift, then your rib cage expand, until your heart lifts … Now exhale in a way that is natural for you, comfortably expelling all the air.

Pause.

Now, we are going to work with the upward and downward flow of energy in your body and the balancing of these energies with your breath. So bring your attention back to your breath and hands once more … When you breathe in, bring your attention to the hand over your navel and when you breathe out, bring your attention to the hand over your heart … Breathing in, your awareness travels to your navel … Breathing out, your awareness moves up to the heart … Breathing in and out, fully, easily, and effortlessly … feeling your breath flow deep within … going downward as you breathe in and rising as you breathe out.

Now, imagine that there is an interior chamber, a chamber of light extending from deep within the heart right down to below the navel. It's deep within the core of the body … and as you breathe, a pathway is cleared and illuminated that runs deep within the core of your body.

Continue saturating your interior core with breath … soaking it in and clearing a pathway that glimmers and glows, giving you the internal freedom that breathing gives … Your interior column begins to sparkle and twinkle as your breath feeds your body … fortifying and balancing and harmonizing with the flow of breath.

The column of light glows and radiates, humming with life... and the light begins to expand, becoming spacious until it extends to the top of your head and to the tips of your toes... and fingers... Bask in the experience... Soak it in.

Quite naturally, the radiance automatically begins to go beyond your physical form and outline... illuminating the space around you... feeling and becoming more and more spacious... spreading out and beyond your body.

Pause.

Now, it's time to find a private place inside yourself to safely store this energy... Tuck it in, so it can continue to fortify you and light your way.

Pause.

It's time now to gradually make the transition back... Begin by feeling whatever you are sitting or lying on... getting a sense of its solid strength and stability... Now bring your attention back to your breath and body... and stretch however you like... As you stretch, your body and mind wake up... feeling refreshed and rejuvenated.

Author's note: In yoga, the inhalation is referred to as prana (pronounced PRAH-nah) and has an upward movement associated with it. If you focus on the upward movement while inhaling, a lifting of energy and a light and spacious feeling results. Try it now.

The exhalation is called apana (pronounced ah-PAH-nah) and has a downward movement. If you focus on a downward movement while exhaling, a lowering of energy results along with the feeling of being grounded. Try it now.

On the other hand, a balancing of energies occurs and can be felt if the upward flow (inhalation, prana) is tempered with drawing the awareness down to the navel, and if the downward flow (exhalation, apana) is tempered with drawing the awareness upward to the heart. Try it now.

Guided Imagery
Mental Movies: the Inner Play of the Body, Mind, and Spirit

Imagination is more important than knowledge.

Albert Einstein

Guided imagery, also referred to as creative visualization, is intentional daydreaming. It aims to magnify the positive aspects of the mind-body connection. It elicits genuine relaxation, which awakens and activates the natural ability for self-healing to occur. Guided imagery helps one uncover inner truth and direction while stimulating intuition. Guided imagery helps with changing behaviors and habits. With regular practice, your skill and efficiency will improve and your results will increase.

Guided imagery takes place in a relaxed state that is entered through focused, full, easy, slow breathing. This state can also be elicited through progressive muscular relaxation techniques, taking time to tense and squeeze each muscle and then release the tension. Focused breathing and progressive muscular relaxation prepare the body for guided imagery and creative visualization.

Once relaxed, the mind is guided in a process similar to daydreaming. The difference is that in daydreaming the mind is allowed to go wherever it pleases. Instead of this, the mind is directed in a specific and special manner. For example, a guided imagery exercise might ask you to focus on a setting or environment that feels safe and comfortable. This can be accomplished by mentally seeing the setting, feeling or experiencing the environment, or using the senses of sound or smell. As Belleruth Naparstek says, "there are many right ways to experience guided imagery." Other guided imagery techniques are geared to awakening the intuition or encouraging health and healing.

Don't be surprised if your experience changes each time you repeat a script. It is common for one's own imagination to change and embellish the suggestions. This is a sign that your inborn imagination is guiding you. Allowing this will enable your experience to be more potent.

Normally, imagery that brings out emotion is more effective than imagery that doesn't. Responding emotionally is a good sign that the imagery is working for you in a deep and genuine way.

The visualizations that follow feature imagery based on the elements of earth, water, fire, air, light, and space and will spark your imagination. These elements also relate to the chakras.

Woodland Walk — Element: Earth (15 minutes)

My Garden — Element: Earth (15 minutes)

Magical Sea — Element: Water (12 minutes)

The Fireplace — Element: Fire (12 minutes)

Taking Flight — Element: Air (12 minutes)

The Convertible Ride — Element: Light (10 minutes)

The Hot Air Balloon Ride — Element: Space (12 minutes)

Woodland Walk

Guided Imagery

Element: Earth

Time: 15 minutes

Summary: An enjoyable walk in the woods renews energy and vitality.

Begin by treating yourself to an enjoyable and satisfying stretch. Go ahead, it's time to loosen up and stretch so you can reclaim your energy. That's right. Stretch all over.

Now allow your entire body to settle and relax comfortably ... if your legs or arms are crossed, please uncross them and settle yourself into whatever you are sitting or lying on.

Take in a nice big breath ... fill your lungs full ... and breathe out to let go from deep inside ... And now, simply follow your breath in ... and out ... allowing each breath to refresh you on many levels.

With your eyes closed or barely open, begin to shift your attention away from the world around you to your inner world of sensations and into your imagination. It will do you good.

Take a big breath in ... and sigh it out.

Let your imagination take you out into the woods for an adventure that will help you feel refreshed and more like yourself again ... These woods are quite special ... a place where you can escape and feel safe ... your own private hideaway. Pretend you are there now.

It's the perfect day to be outside ... It's gorgeous and the temperature feels great ... Overhead, the sky is a brilliant blue ... The sunlight surrounds you with healing light and warms you through and through ... The clouds form a multitude of shapes and drift on by, and as the clouds come and go, your worries evaporate ... and your mind clears, like the depth and expanse of the infinite sky ... The trees are magnificent and the woods are brimming with life ... It smells delightful.

Pause.

Imagine yourself walking along a path... take a little time and notice what it's like... How wide is it?... What is it made of?... How does it feel to be walking on it?

With each step you take, notice how you feel more and more alive with a bounce in your step... It's hard not to smile. Walking feels effortless and invigorating... like you're gliding upon a magic carpet. Walking along, your tiredness melts away, and more and more you notice feeling renewed and revived with boundless energy. There's a spring in your step, and it feels great to be here.

Looking around, notice your surroundings... There are many types of trees... all different shapes and sizes, each one inspiring in its own special way... and perhaps there's a rainbow of smiling wildflowers dancing in the light... The smell of the woods comes alive.

Notice the sounds that come and go... Perhaps you hear the sound of a gentle breeze rustling through the leaves... the songs of the birds... or an occasional bark of a dog, off in the distance... What other sounds can you notice?

The sunlight streams through, beaming a golden light that dapples through the branches above... casting shadows here and there... The air tingles and the woods sparkle with life... It feels radiant, and the fresh air renews your energy with each and every breath. Take a few moments to continue down your path, walking along at a comfortable pace, following your curiosity and losing yourself in the sounds, the smells, and the colors all around.

Pause.

You become aware of the distant sound of tumbling water. It sparks your curiosity as to where it's coming from... It might even be a waterfall... so you take off in a new direction, not sure what you'll find... Lo and behold, you discover a beautiful creek that is gurgling and chuckling by... The water cascades constantly over the rocks like a dance... and the water's surface glimmers and glows... If you wish, you may dip into the refreshing stream of water... It feels exhilarating... and you feel invigorated with energy... Relishing each and every moment... you are reminded that this very creek gradually flows into the river that eventually joins the oceans of the earth.

Pause.

Back on the path again, notice how the canopy of trees is protective and comforting and how the leaves whisper in the soft breeze.... The sunlight sparkles through, bringing its warmth and wonder to everything it shines upon, and you drink in its beauty ... soaking its magic into your heart of hearts.

And now you become aware that there's a clearing up ahead ... As you enter you feel a hushed silence ... The clearing is carpeted in softness ... and feels magical and enchanted.

Take some time to explore this special place ... How large is it? ... What do you notice in the horizon? ... What is the air like? ... What plants and animals are present?

Pause.

Now your attention is captured with watching the squirrels and rabbits darting about ... noticing the birds flying and hopping from place to place, singing their songs ... and noticing all the other wildlife at work and at play.

Pause.

Notice how boundless energy begins surging through you so you feel like joining in all the activity ... feeling the urge to enjoy yourself and play, just like the animals. So, imagine enjoying yourself, having fun, exploring, discovering, and playing ... Perhaps you'd like to fly like a bird or climb a tree like a raccoon and be carefree.

Off in the distance, you notice a special place that has a hammock ... and a park bench ... and a swing ... you glide on over and settle into one or the other for a while ... enjoying yourself completely and allowing yourself to daydream.

Pause.

You notice now that an animal is trying to get your attention ... What is it? ... What details do you notice? ... It's coming closer ... and you're getting excited ... You can tell that it has a gift or perhaps a message just for you ... And that's what happens, you are given a personal gift or a message from this special animal.

Pause.

And now, you'd like to give something back in return.

Pause.

From this extraordinary space, you begin feeling lighter and more free and easy, feeling the surge of life pulsing through you ... replenishing your energy...Each time you breathe, you can tell you are being completely restored from deep inside, from an unending and powerful source of energy and vitality...and you feel your energy and enthusiasm pouring back to you. So continue on with courage and a willingness to trust, knowing you can more than handle what's ahead with a knowing confidence.

Having come full circle now, it's time to return from your woodland walk...noticing how your energy and resourcefulness has grown and expanded...and knowing you can come back, again and again...and each time you do, your experience will deepen and grow...

Whenever you're ready, you can begin to stretch and move...feeling full of life, alert and ready for whatever comes next.

Recorded on *Wholesome Energizers* CD by Julie Lusk with music by Tom Laskey. Available from Whole Person Associates at 800-247-6789 or on the Web at wholeperson.com.

My Garden

Guided Imagery and Affirmations

Time: 15 minutes

Summary: Using guided imagery and affirmations; a garden scene is created for cultivating qualities to reclaim health, inner vitality and energy.

The mind becomes clear and serene when
the qualities of the heart are cultivated.

Yoga Sutra 1.33

Stretch comfortably and move around so you can settle down and feel comfortable... Take a big breath in... and sigh it out.

Be still for a few moments and let go of muscular tightness and tension... feeling your body softening into the comfort of relaxation... simply, letting go of muscular tension... and breathing in a way that is slow, smooth, and deep... taking your time to breathe all the way in... and all the way out. Doing so, in and of itself, will release tension and replace it with needed energy.

And now, as you breathe slowly and smoothly, allow your awareness to expand, making room for your imagination and for positive affirmations, used to reclaim your health, inner strength, and energy.

Imagine that your life is like a garden... a unique garden... In this garden, you can plant qualities and traits that will help you along your way and give you the energy and inspiration you need. So it's a garden of life that is worthwhile and one where you know you belong.

Let's explore your garden... going there now in your mind's eye... noticing what it's like... how it looks... how it smells... and sounds... What shape is it in?... What's already growing?... What's waiting to be planted?... What's ready to be weeded away?

Notice that place you've always wanted to cultivate and nurture, perhaps a place where it's hard for things to grow, where something extra is needed, but you aren't sure what it is.

And, into this place, imagine getting ready to plant those qualities that can help you along your way...qualities that encourage and inspire, bringing you the vitality and confidence to be faithful to your true nature...Perhaps they're qualities such as health...quiet courage...acceptance...wisdom...joy...or others that are meaningful to you.

Pause.

Imagine planting those qualities now...in just the right amounts...and right where they're needed...Go ahead with your planting...placing each quality with confidence and trust.

Pause.

Giving them what they need to grow and develop.

Pause.

And now feel how they are taking root...and notice them growing...into your garden of life and living.

Pause.

Along with what you've already planted, you can now plant your ideas, your wishes, and your dreams...things you'd like to create and see happen in your life...becoming aware of what's it going to take...the actions and resources and support needed for your dreams to come true.

Pause.

And now, imagine yourself going forward, jumping ahead into the future...Experience it happening...and watch as your dreams come true.

Another area in your garden needs to be thinned and could use some weeding...so spend some time taking away those things, those distractions, that are slowing you down or causing you to get sidetracked.

Pause.

Imagine removing whatever it is and putting the weeds, those things that are getting in your way, into the compost heap where they can change and transform into fertilizer that will help you with your new growth.

Perhaps there's something that needs your attention...something that it's time to complete or release...so your energy can be freed and you can move on.

There's another place in your garden where there's a fountain...Imagine what this fountain is like...what it's made of...how it's flowing...how it sounds...As you gaze at your fountain, you discover, more and more, that it becomes one that feeds and fills you with energy and inspiration... enjoying how your fountain is free to flow and how it is so refreshing... bringing you vitality and stimulating your inspiration... as the water splashes and dances.

Now that you have done some planting and weeding, it's time to step back so you can watch over your garden... knowing that for your garden to grow and flourish, it needs just the right amount of care and attention from inside yourself, as well as from outside influences. Your life, just like a garden, needs a balance of sunshine, rain, and fertilizer... darkness and light... And somehow, and from somewhere, there's an inner knowing you have, from your heart of hearts, that gives you just the right balance of effort, and letting go, and letting it be, to thrive and succeed.

Each time you return to your garden and listen once again, you can check on what's been planted... you can do more planting and weeding so your garden of life is a place where you want to be... a place where you belong... a garden where you always feel welcome.

And finally, it's time to use a few affirmations and the power of your mind and intention to help you move along. Allow the following statements to echo in your mind, perhaps, repeating them to yourself, silently, or aloud... letting them move through you, refreshing and renewing you... and allowing them to soak in deep inside... If an affirmation doesn't seem to fit you, don't worry, just breathe slowly and softly, and wait for the next one... or change it to suit yourself, just so it's still positive... or simply pretend that it's true.

In my garden of life...

I am wholesome and healthy in body, mind, and spirit.

I have strength and courage.

I feel peace and contentment.

I receive acceptance and support.

I feel love and affection.

Continue on your own, planting qualities and affirmations that are especially meaningful to you... When you're ready, stretch, open your eyes, and enjoy feeling refreshed and energized. Remember these qualities throughout the day and watch as they show up and grow.

Recorded on *Wholesome Energizers* CD by Julie Lusk with music by Tom Laskey. Available from Whole Person Associates at 800-247-6789 or on the Web at wholeperson.com.

Magical Sea

Guided Imagery

Element: Water

Time: 12 minutes

Summary: A trip to the water's edge is refreshing and brings about new insights.

◑ ◑ ◑

Allow your entire body to relax comfortably... settling yourself into whatever you are sitting or lying on... allowing your muscles to relax and soften... Take a big breath in... and sigh it out.

Breathe in a way that feels free and easy... slowly breathing in... and out... in... and out... relaxing further into the steady rhythm of your breath... When your mind wanders, simply bring your attention to the steady stream of your breath... sending any tightness, discomfort or tension out with your breath. This is a time for you to let go of stress and strain, to enjoy your imagination through guided imagery, and to feel wholesome.

Each time you breathe out, pause a moment... then when you're ready for more air, breathe in... resting in the quiet space between breaths.

Pause.

Let your imagination drift to being outside... out in the open... Imagine yourself along your favorite shore at the water's edge... The shore is sandy and glistens in the sunlight... You notice rocks and stones of all sizes and shapes and colors... The shells are magnificent and strewn all about... Allow your awareness to roam, exploring where you are.

Walking along, let your footsteps sink comfortably into the sand, step by step... Take in the sights, notice the colors... the time of day... Take in all the richness of the scenery... it's beautiful and inspiring... See the shining color of the water and how the light sparkles on it.

If you'd like, shift your attention to all the sounds... listen to the waves as they flow in and out... It's melodic and rhythmic and soothing... ... and be aware of other sounds, like the birds... the breeze.

As the surf comes in to the shore, the water's foam makes waves and patterns in the sand...Gaze as the waves go in and out, watching the swirling patterns of the water and the sand...going to and fro.

Perhaps you'd like to enjoy the aromas and fragrances at the water's edge...the clean and crisp air...scents of the plant life...What else do you notice? Let your imagination embellish your experience.

Pause.

The sun's rays are streaming down and shining...Feel the sun's gentle warmth...It wraps you in cozy comforting healing.

Now, your attention is drawn to the sky...Watch how the feathery clouds float and form new fluffy shapes...and how they slowly dissolve and form new creations.

And now, gaze beyond the clouds into the expanse of the clear sky...marveling at the colors of the sky...It looks so clear, and the air is crisp and refreshing...Become conscious of its spaciousness...stretching out beyond infinity.

Feel or watch yourself pick up a stick and feel its weight and dampness in your hands...Begin drawing or writing something in the sand that represents your worries and concerns...or simply begin digging a hole in the sand to bury your troubles.

Pause.

And now a wave comes in and washes all your worries away, taking them all away...Each time the waves come and go, you feel freer and lighter...The coming and going of the waves is calming and soothing...hearing the sound of the waves in the background and feeling the atmosphere in the air.

Pause.

As you continue your walk, feel your feet sink briefly with each step...and notice the multi-colored shells in the sand...In the distance, you see a very special one that stands out from all the others, and you walk toward it and pick it up, noticing its shape...its size...and its color...enjoying what you've found. Slowly, the shell begins to sparkle and glow, and you notice that it's magical...You're awed at its uniqueness and character.

Something tells you that the shell has a hidden message inside that will help you in some way...This message can appear as a word or phrase, an image or a sound...All you have to do is focus your awareness inside...as

you do, something will occur to you that can help you ... Take a few moments for this special source of insight and wisdom to reveal itself.

Pause.

You can either toss it back or save this magical shell in a safe place ... any
place, just so it's safe.

Begin bringing your attention back to your breath ... gently focusing
your attention on the rise and fall of your breath, like the waves ... As
you breathe in more fully, you feel yourself becoming more alert and
awake ... It's a special feeling of being calm, relaxed and alert ... Continuing to breathe, you feel a surge of energy pulsing through you, feeling
fully alive ... When you're ready, you can stretch, enjoying the movement of your body ... And open your eyes feeling uplifted and ready to
take on your next activity.

Recorded on *Wholesome Relaxation* CD by Julie Lusk with music by
Tom Laskey. Available from Whole Person Associates at 800-247-6789
or on the Web at wholeperson.com.

The Fireplace

Guided Imagery

Element: Fire

Time: 12 minutes

Summary: Experience the comfort of sitting by the fire in a cozy room.

Begin by treating yourself to an enjoyable and satisfying stretch. Go ahead, it's time to loosen up and stretch so you can reclaim your energy. That's right. Stretch all over.

And now, allow your entire body to settle and relax comfortably ... if your legs or arms are crossed, uncross them and settle yourself into whatever you are sitting or lying on.

Take a big breath in ... and sigh it out.

Take in a few more nice big breaths ... fill your lungs full ... and breathe out to let go from deep inside.

And now, simply follow your natural breath in ... and out ... allowing each breath to restore you on many levels.

Pause.

With your eyes closed or barely open, begin to shift your attention away from the world around you to your inner world of sensations and into your imagination. It will do you good.

Take another big breath in ... and sigh it out.

Imagine being in a cozy room ... one that feels homey and comforting to you ... perhaps a room you know ... perhaps not ... as long as it's cozy and comforting to you ... a place where you feel welcome and safe, just as you are.

In your mind's eye, experience this room in whatever way you want ... using whatever senses you can ... Some people can visualize and "see" things in their mind's eye; many others don't. It doesn't matter, just so long as you can bring the essence of a cozy, comforting room into your imagination ... Can you feel what it's like to be there? ... Or maybe it's easier to notice how it looks... or the aromas... or the sounds... that take you to a cozy and comfortable room in your mind's eye to bring it alive.

Take a few moments for yourself to explore... and to discover, more and more, a room that brings you peace and comfort... Simply, experience this room in a natural, easy way... discovering a place where you can be settled and undisturbed.

This room contains some of your favorite things... Allow your imagination the freedom to notice your favorite things in this special room.

Pause.

In your mind's eye, you notice an area that you hadn't been aware of... In this area you become aware of a crackling fire in a fireplace... What is it like for you?... Is the fire large or small... Is it burning brightly... or are the embers merely glowing?

Pause.

Now, notice a chair that is there just for you... Sink into it... and it forms around you, taking a shape that supports you... Settle into this comfortable chair, in the cozy room, by the fireplace... basking in the experience.

Now allow your awareness to return to the fire in the fireplace... notice how it has changed, as all fires do... Gazing into the fire... observe the flames... the warmth... the unique light... the smell of burning wood.

Taking care of it... tending it, if needed.

You're mesmerized by the experience of being in a cozy room, surrounded by comfort... gazing at the fireplace... savoring it.

Pause.

> Ur attn. is pulled toward _____ B- this is ur space, time.

Now your attention is drawn to the window... Looking out, notice what it's like outside... No matter what the weather, you're safe, warm, and comfortable inside your place of comfort.

So up / u
toner p/u
U. F Ses'd
to note stress
6... watching
then dissolve int
the flame
(just as
thoughts come
go...

Pause.

If you like, you can invite someone to join you, or you can be by yourself... going with whatever occurs to you... Simply go with it for a while... wherever your imagination goes.

Pause.

Now the time has come to leave, knowing you can return, using your mind's eye to return ... knowing this is a place that's inside you ... But for now, take a few minutes to end your experience of being by the fire ... in a place of comfort and safety.

Bring your attention back to the place where you are ... and when you're ready, begin stretching. Wake your body and mind with a stretch ... Open your eyes and be here now.

Taking Flight

Guided Imagery

Element: Air

Time: 12 minutes.

Summary: Experience the joy of flying like a bird and feeling gratitude for the air and wind.

🕊 🕊 🕊

Allow your entire body to relax comfortably... settling yourself into whatever you are sitting or lying on... allowing your muscles to relax and soften.

Take a big breath in... and sigh it out.

Take in another big breath, and when you exhale, feel free to send it out with a sounding sigh... relieving more and more tension with each exhalation.

Now, breathe in a way that feels free and easy... slowly breathing in... and out... in... and out... relaxing further into the steady rhythm of your breath... When your mind wanders, simply bring your attention to the steady stream of your breath... sending any tightness, discomfort or tension out with your breath. This is a time for you to let go of stress and strain, to enjoy your imagination through guided imagery.

Each time you breathe out, pause a moment... then when you're ready for more air, breathe in... and rest in the quiet space between breaths.

Pause.

Imagine being outdoors in a wide, open space... a space where the air is crisp and refreshing... Imagine a breeze blowing... feeling its touch against your skin... Perhaps you notice it blowing through your hair... In your mind's eye, notice how the wind comes and goes... feeling stronger at times... and calming down... alternating between gusts of breeze... and quieting down.

Notice the quality of the air... Is it moist... or dry?... Is it warm... or cool?

Can you tune into the sounds of the breeze as it moves all around?

The air and the wind are vital to everything living on planet earth. The wind circulates the air and serves an important purpose in the fertilization of plants...It contains moisture and is vital in the making of rain, and moving clouds...The wind brings us water from the oceans and oxygen from the rain forests...and the land and the wind serve a valuable role in heating and cooling the air that surrounds us.

Acknowledge the importance of the wind and its presence in your own way.

Pause.

Once again, imagine being in an open space outside...a place where you can see the depth and expanse of the wide open sky...and notice the birds flying through the sky...soaring gracefully...flapping their wings at times...and gliding elegantly on the air currents.

Pause.

Bring to mind one of your favorite flying birds...and notice its glorious color...its size...and other characteristics of this bird.

Pause.

Out of the blue, you can magically experience your surroundings from the birds' perspective...and you are now able to see with keen awareness, way off into the distance...and you can even see all around you, not just in front.

And just like a bird, your hearing has changed...and you are paying attention to sounds in a whole new way.

Begin to feel what it's like to have a body like a bird...and become aware of having feathers and wings...legs and a beak.

Imagine flying through the air...flapping your wings to take you up into the sky...and rising up on a warm current of air...a thermal that naturally lifts you upward so you can enjoy flying effortlessly...soaring...and gliding...flying higher...and higher still...coasting through the clouds...and back out into the sunshine...simply enjoying the freedom of flight with utter abandonment and joy.

Pause.

For a while, you pause and perch in a tree, way up above everything else...watching the other wildlife, way up in the trees...watching the other birds... hearing their songs and their twittering... noticing the activity of the squirrels and other animals... way up in the trees... Perhaps you'd like to fly from branch to branch like an acrobat... exploring your surroundings, more and more... Because your eyes and ears are now so powerful, you're able to experience your world in a whole new way.

Pause.

It's time now to fly down from the tree and through the air again... feeling the winds lift you for a while... and artfully swoop down... soaring all around.

And now it's time to descend through the air... past the treetops... and finally onto the ground... As you land, your experience of being like a bird is transformed back into being yourself again... except there's a part of you that feels exuberant and full of delight.

Bring your attention back to where you are sitting or lying down... and the place where you are... and when you're ready, begin stretching, waking up your body and mind with a stretch... Open your eyes and be here now.

Repeat the above instructions until everyone is alert.

Author's note: Special thanks to Julia Young and Janet Chahrour for their inspiration.

The Convertible Ride

Guided Imagery

Element: Light

Time: 10 minutes

Summary: Experience the joy of going for a ride in a convertible and enjoy the sunlight along with all the other scenery.

Stretch comfortably and move around so you can settle down and feel comfortable on whatever you are sitting or lying on ... Take a big breath in ... and sigh it out.

Be still for a few moments and let go of muscular tightness and tension ... feeling your body softening into the comfort of relaxation ... simply letting go of muscular tension. When you notice pockets of tension, try tightening those muscles even more, hold for a moment, and then release completely. Practice this until you feel the muscular tension dissolving and going away.

Allow your breathing to become slow, smooth, and even ... taking your time to breathe all the way in ... and all the way out. Doing so, in and of itself, will release tension and replace it with needed energy.

And now, as you breathe slowly and smoothly, allow your imagination to enlarge and, using your mind's eye, imagine a convertible car ... Become aware of its color ... and make ... Is it old or brand new? ... What does the interior look like?

Like magic, someone hands you the keys and invites you to go for a leisurely and fun ride ... alone or with friends.

Imagine yourself getting in ... Sink into the seat ... and turn the key ... The motor springs to life. You hear the hum of the engine ... and you feel a smile radiating from deep inside yourself and cheering you.

You take off in your convertible ... It's a beautiful day ... and you feel the warm rays of the sun on your skin ... At the same time, the wind keeps you cool ... It's a perfect combination of warmth from the sun and the coolness of the refreshing air ... cruising along in your convertible.

All at once, you are driving along a country road...It's a winding road with gentle curves...and rolling hills...and the car hugs the road as you cruise along...taking the curves and the hills with ease.

Around the next curve, there's a wide-open expanse with crops growing on both sides of the road...You notice the sun streaming down and remember that the sun is the source of light that is vital for all life.

Up ahead, a roadside stand overflows with an abundance of fruit and vegetables. You come to a stop, get out, and stretch your legs, gazing at the abundance of fresh fruit and vegetables...Everything imaginable is at your fingertips...so you admire the ripe plums...the golden apricots...the crisp, juicy apples...the luscious berries...and all the other fruits.

There are also many vegetables...fresh corn...an assortment of tomatoes...and all the green vegetables. Imagine getting something to eat and enjoying it to the fullest.

Now hop back into the car and take off again...cruising the countryside...with the top down...feeling free...and having fun. The light of the sun highlights the scenery...bringing everything to life...so much so that everything seems to be glowing.

Around the next bend you see a herd of animals out in the field...and you drive for miles and miles...noticing the animal life...and the landscape.

As the sun begins to fade, the clouds start to move in until it gets almost dark...The next thing you know, you feel a few raindrops so you instantly put the top up, just in time because the rain starts pelting down...but you don't care because you're protected and safe with the top up.

Pause.

Off in the distance, you see the sky clearing...You continue driving and the sun peeks out...getting brighter and brighter...and so you put the top back down. The air is fresher than ever before, and all at once, there's a magnificent rainbow...It's huge and glorious, and its beauty is breathtaking...Your car travels through the light of the rainbow...First there's red, the most gorgeous shade of red you've ever seen. It bursts into streaming fireworks, lighting everything up...Now there's a brilliant orange light that you can almost taste, and it radiates its orange color in all directions...and next a golden yellow that shines brightly, beautifying everything it comes in contact with, twinkling and glowing...It's as if you can swim through all the colors... The green light sparkles and feels full of life... The blue glows, and bubbles into all other shades of blue... The purple shimmers and glistens and transforms into swirls of different tones of purple and violet... Then it grows fainter until it's a clear white light, clean and refreshing, like freshly fallen snow... and it occurs to you to make a wish.

Pause.

Again you're aware of riding in your convertible. You notice a knob that you hadn't noticed before. If you use it, it will magically transport you to anywhere in the world you would like to go... so imagine yourself being transported to wherever you would like to be.

Pause.

It's time now to come back from your convertible ride... so imagine returning with a renewed sense of adventure and freedom. When you're ready, stretch and open your eyes.

Hot Air Balloon Ride

Guided Imagery

Element: Space

Time: 12 minutes

Summary: Enjoy an uplifting adventure on a hot air balloon ride to gain a new perspective and to feel open, free, and spacious.

◍ ◍ ◍

Take time by preparing yourself for an imaginary adventure designed to be uplifting and to allow you to feel open, free and spacious.

But first, it's important to take a few moments to get connected to your inner sense of being centered and wholesome.

Breathe in fully, feeling yourself expand... then breath out and allow yourself to let go... breathing in slowly and fully, expanding... and breathing out, letting go... Each time you breathe out, let go of tension, be it physical tension... mental chatter... or perhaps emotional commotion... letting it all soften and dissolve, each time you let your breath go... to empty yourself of stress... and strain.

As tension releases and evaporates, notice how you're feeling more and more at ease... more and more settled inside... by releasing tension and replacing it with feeling free... more and more free, with each breath... so that for a while, you can be free of your worries and troubles... Your mindful breathing opens the way to being open and free... to feeling an inner freshness... and an openness.

To enlarge this openness even more, call to mind something that reminds you of feeling free and easy... letting your imagination take you right there now... to a time or a place or a circumstance that opens you up in a way that is natural and feels safe for you.

Pause.

In your mind's eye, imagine a hot air balloon off in the distance... From your vantage point, notice the balloon and its colors... a multitude of colors that are beautiful to you... any colors... just so they're pleasing to you... Open your imagination and let the colors flood in.

You're inspired now to go for a ride in the hot air balloon ... Approaching the basket, notice how well it's made ... the clever way it's designed ... and been made ready to take you on an adventure ... an uplifting and fun-filled adventure.

Climbing aboard, a rush of excitement runs through you, anticipating what's ahead ... In a whoosh, you're off, taking off ... lifting up ... going higher and higher at a comfortable pace for you ... noticing the air and how fresh and clean it is, as you rise up in the hot air balloon.

And now, take a few moments to toss your concerns over the side and notice how they disintegrate into nothingness ... As this happens, a lightness of being occurs.

Pause.

As the hot air balloon continues on, the view of the landscape below changes. As you go higher, what's down below looks smaller ... and smaller ... Going higher, the land and water below looks like swatches of color ... green strips of the trees and forests ... rivers like ribbons intertwining and flowing into the huge expanse of the oceans ... Cities and towns take on a brand new perspective ... Clouds hover over some areas, casting shadows below ... and you enjoy the play of light and shadows as natural shifts and changes take place.

Here's a special pair of binoculars that can help you see. They'll enable you to zoom in on whatever interests you with crystal clarity. Use them to explore the world beneath you.

Pause.

From this vantage point, the air is pure and refreshing ... and clean ... and fills you full ... giving you balance ... and harmony ... and contentment.

Somehow, the balloon continues to lift you higher into the sky and atmosphere until you are safely soaring among the planets and stars. The planet earth appears as a globe suspended in space, orbiting around the sun ... and the earth looks sun-kissed.

You're feeling really free and can appreciate and enjoy the expansiveness that extends on and on and on ... expanding way above, below, and all around ... into forever ... and this awareness touches and awakens a place in you that is spacious and expansive ... a place that welcomes you, enabling you to realize a new perspective as you float along in the heavens ... This heavenly feeling resonates inside you ... and you can merge with it ... in a way that feels right to you.

Pause.

After a while, it's time to return to planet earth...As you descend, the oceans and forests and cities are once again recognizable, becoming clearer and clearer...gaining in size until you are able to hover a bit, observing the places and people below you...from a new viewpoint and with a new outlook.

Pause.

Now it's time to touch back down. The hot air balloon lands...and you notice the solid ground that's been waiting for you...Before stepping out of the ballon, take time to savor your experience in your own way.

Pause.

When you're ready, you'll open your eyes and stretch, and your mind will awaken and become alert.

Healing Guided Imagery

*When disturbed by negative feelings and thoughts,
cultivate the positive.*

Yoga Sutras 2.33

Healing imagery is a powerful way to increase your sense of well-being. Studies have shown that it reduces stress levels and will likely improve your health. Your mind will clear, your emotions will settle, your body will relax, and your heart and spirit will open. Guided imagery is widely used in hospitals, wellness centers, religious settings, and mental health clinics.

Brain Refresher (5 minutes or longer)

Cultivate the Positive: Pratipaksha Bhavana (10 minutes or longer)

Prana Hands: Prana Dharana (15 minutes or longer)

The Pond of Love (10 to 12 minutes)

Liquid Blue Healing (10 minutes)

Cruising... Magical Motorcycle Rider (15 minutes)

Intuition Time (8 minutes)

Brain Refresher

Guided Meditation

Contributed by Lilias Folan

Time: 5 minutes or longer

Summary: Refresh your brain with the sound of N. This method can also be used with the bija and vowel sounds that are found on the chakra chart. Simply direct the appropriate sound to the area of the body associated with each chakra.

❂ ❂ ❂

Sit tall in a chair or on a meditation cushion. Part your lips slightly and relax your jaw. Place your tongue as if to pronounce the letter "N."

Close your eyes and on your next exhale, tone a long NNN sound, keeping your facial muscles soft ... Focus your attention on the sound ... Follow it through until the very end.

Comfortably breathe in ... again slowly exhale ... Aim the NNN sound upwards into your brain ... Feel the vibrations in your eyes ... Follow the sound until its end.

Comfortably breathe in ... This time, play with the tone ... soft ... medium ... loud ... high ... higher.

Imagine the sound sending waves of refreshing vibrations to every cell of your good friend, your brain.

Repeat three to five more times. Then sit quietly.

Bring a little smile upon your lips ... dive inward ... feel awake and clear ... and enjoy the stillness.

If a thought comes ... let it float on through.

Stay and enjoy the stillness for a little longer.

Author's note: Lilias, America's best-known yoga teacher, has inspired millions of people for years with her PBS television series, *Lilias! Yoga and You.* Lilias leads workshops nationally and internationally and is a major presenter at yoga conferences. Friendly, caring, and down-to-earth, she teaches yoga in Cincinnati, Ohio, and shares her love of it in many books, videos and CDs. Go to liliasyoga.com for more information.

Cultivate the Positive
Pratipaksha Bhavana

When disturbed by negative thoughts and feelings, cultivate the positive.
                                                    Yoga Sutra 2.33

Healing Practice

Pratipaksha Bhavana is pronounced Prah-tee-pak-shah Bhah-van-ah

Time: 10 minutes or longer

Summary: Pratipaksha Bhavana is a meditation practice that teaches us to exchange negative thoughts and feelings for positive ones. This nurtures our capacity to react constructively and mindfully in a level-headed and calm manner to people and situations and makes us less likely to react automatically and negatively.

Many breathing exercises teach us to breathe in the positive and breathe out the negative. Not so with Pratipaksha Bhavana. In this practice, we breathe in and out the positive to counteract the negative. This emphasizes helpful qualities, enabling them to take root quickly and efficiently. In the former practice, we take one step forward and two steps back because more attention is placed on the negative (due to naturally breathing out longer) with less time on the positive. In fact, the unwanted qualities are right before us ready and waiting to be breathed back in.

Pratipaksha Bhavana can also literally change one thought or feeling for another. When someone is unkind and behaves badly, or when you are tempted to be critical, choose to focus on the positive instead. It's similar to the carpenter who drives out the old nail with a new one.

Begin by closing your eyes... bringing your attention to your breath. Spend some time focusing your attention on your ongoing breath. You may wish to say silently to yourself "I know I'm breathing in" on the inhalation, and "I know I'm breathing out" on the exhalation. Continue on until you feel a settling inside. Take your time with this process of settling yourself down.

As your mind wanders, gently return your awareness to your breath.

Choose a negative thought or feeling that you would like to transform into something positive. At first, start with something that is mild, something somewhat irritating, instead of going right into the core problems of your life... so you can get used to the practice gradually, and in stages... Possibilities include worry, fear, sadness, or being critical. As always, what you want to work with is up to you.

Choose something now that is bothersome to you.

Instead of holding on to the negative or trying to push it away... let it go... set it free... let it melt away like honey in hot tea... let it dissolve.

Pause.

Now think of what this negative's positive counterpart would be. For example, you could exchange strength for worry, happiness for sadness, or understanding for a critical attitude.

Take a few moments to think of a virtue that you would like to replace the negative with.

Bring your attention back to your breath. While breathing in, you could say, "Breathing in, I am (name the new virtue)," and while breathing out, you could say "Breathing out, I am (name the virtue)."

Pause.

Now call to mind something that reminds you of the trait you are developing and nurturing. This could be a person, a place, an object, or image. Focus your attention on it, dwelling in the memory or experience of it.

Pause.

Every time your attention wanders, bring your attention back to the positive and return to cultivating it.

Pause.

To strengthen your experience, see or sense yourself in a situation or circumstance responding with the new characteristic you are working with.

Pause.

Return your attention to the positive virtue and welcome it inward.

Remember and reflect on the positive often. Each time you are given an opportunity, practice.

When you are ready, open your eyes and stretch.

Prana Hands
Prana Dharana

Healing Practice

Prana Dharana is pronounced PRAH-nah DAH-ra-nah

Time: 15 minutes or longer

Summary: Prana Dharana can be found in the Upanishads, teachings spanning back 5000 years. It is the technique of projecting the life force (prana) into specific parts of the body in order to restore health. Ancient sages claimed it would conquer all illnesses and fatigue. Prana Hands is an example of Prana Dharana. For Prana Hands to be most effective, it must be done extremely slowly, almost as if you are moving in a dream.

Focus your attention into the moment.

Place your hands together in front of your heart in the prayer position with your fingers and palms touching each other. Press your hands together and begin breathing deep Ujjayi and Dirgha breaths.

Press and rub your hands together in very small movements until they begin to feel very warm to awaken and activate the healing energy.

Pause.

Very, very slowly, begin separating your hands until the skin is barely touching. Firmly, press them back together. Repeat this process until you notice a growing sensation between your palms, fingers, and fingertips.

Next, slowly begin to separate your hands until they are about three to six inches apart and breathe deeply for a few breaths. You may feel warmth, tingly sensations, pulsations, or even a magnetic attraction between your hands.

Press them firmly together again.

Continue drawing your hands toward and away from each other while sensing the prana like a pillow of energy that sometimes attracts and sometimes presses away. Occasionally rub your palms slowly together again. Gradually move your hands farther and farther away while still feeling the "magnetism."

Once you are in consistent contact with the energy sensations, begin to lift your hands and arms very, very slowly and turn your hands toward your face and eyes without touching physically. Slowly, continue to slowly raise and lower your hands a few inches at a time. Notice any sensations that play across your face.

Now, focus your attention on the part of your body that is in need of healing. Breathe steadily and move your hands in triple slow motion to the place in need. Allow your palms to hover a few inches over the desired area while focusing your attention on the sensation of healing energy between your hands and body.

Let yourself go into your breath and the sensations and focus your attention on the healing energy between your hands and your body. Relax deeply and allow your hands to pulse slowly toward and away from the area in focus while visualizing the flow of healing energy. Healing can occur physically, emotionally, and energetically.

Every now and then, magnify the healing energy by slowly rubbing or pressing your hands together. Hover your hands back over the same area or over another area.

When you are ready to finish, allow your hands to turn toward your heart, the source of healing and pause for a few breaths.

Author's note: Warm thanks to Christopher Baxter for his ideas and help with Prana Hands.

The Pond of Love

Guided Imagery

Time: 10 to 12 minutes

Summary: Enjoy sitting beside a pond that radiates love. Endless variations can result by substituting different characteristics and virtues radiating from the pond. For instance, the pond may be full of peace, understanding or forgiveness. You may also let the participants choose the characteristics on their own by leaving it open-ended. Be creative.

Begin by giving yourself a delightful and satisfying stretch. Go ahead, it's time to loosen up and stretch so you feel better. That's right. Stretch all over.

Now allow your entire body to settle and relax comfortably... If your legs or arms are crossed, uncross them and settle yourself into whatever you are sitting or lying on.

Take in a few nice big breaths... Each time, fill your lungs full... and breathe out to let go from deep inside.

And now, simply follow your instinctive breath in ... and out ... allowing each breath to restore you on many levels.

With your eyes closed or barely open, begin to shift your attention away from the world around you to your inner world of sensations and into your imagination. It will do you good.

Take another big breath in ... and let go.

Imagine that you are sitting beside a secluded pond... It's private... There is nothing to disturb you... Look around... Take in your surroundings... What season is it? ... What colors do you see? ... Do you notice any smells? ... Simply take in the scenery.

Now, direct your attention to the pond... As you look at the pond, you realize that it is not an ordinary pond of water, but a pond filled full of love... Feel love's energy radiating from the pond.

Drawn towards the pond, see yourself coming closer to the water...attracted by the pond, which is radiating love...Look into the depth of the pond...It's full of love...See a beautiful mist hovering above the pond...Notice that the mist is made of love...Breathe it in...It's fulfilling and satisfying...Each time you breathe in, feel the essence of love...surrounding and enfolding you...calming and satisfying...Breathing in, feel the love filtering in and entering your being...smell it...feel it...bringing the love into your being.

Now you notice a boat beside the pond...floating on the pond of love...sweet and pure love...see yourself approaching the boat...getting on board the boat...floating on the pond of love, sweet and pure love...rocking gently, being fully supported by love.

Feel yourself reaching out towards the pond...the pond full of love...Splash the love upon you...Feel it soak into you...filling you with love...Allow it to enter the quiet center of your being...deep within you...in your own special center...your inner most core radiates with love...Feel the love in your center growing...expanding...throughout your entire body...radiating out from your center...circulating through and through.

There may be an area of your life...physically...mentally...emotionally...spiritually...that could benefit from being bathed in love...Feel the love go to that area...bathing you...washing over you...becoming a part of you...Feel the love.

If you like, you may now send this loving feeling to other people...to other places...to other relationships.

Pause.

Bring your attention back to sitting beside the pond...feeling the love.

Pause.

And now return your attention to the present...Begin stretching and moving whenever you are ready...and open your eyes.

Author's note: The Pond of Love is from *30 Scripts for Relaxation, Imagery and Inner Healing, Volume Two* and is recorded on *Refreshing Journeys* by Julie Lusk. Both the book and the recording are available from Whole Person Associates. Call 800-247-6789 or visit wholeperson.com.

Liquid Blue Healing

Healing Guided Imagery

Contributed by Lynne Greene

Time: 10 minutes

Summary: Feel stress, tension, aches, and pain drain away with the help of a healing blue liquid.

◍ ◍ ◍

Allow your body weight to release against the surface supporting it... With each exhalation, allow your body to relax a little more deeply.

Imagine that your body is filled with a warm, blue, healing liquid... This liquid has the power to wash away stress, release chronic tension, and soothe any aches and pains that you may have.

Visualize half of this warm, blue liquid pooling in your belly... Allow it to release and wash away chronic tension held in your abdomen... Feel the liquid wash around your hips... and settle in your low back... Knots are gently washed away.

Allow the liquid to slowly stream into your thighs, washing around your knees... and then let this liquid flow into your lower legs, easing and dissolving pain... The warm, blue liquid gradually flows into your feet and trickles into each toe... When you are ready, allow this liquid to drain out of your toes, taking with it anything that you are ready and willing to let go of.

The other half of this warm, blue liquid is floating peacefully in your head... still and calm like the smooth surface of a lake... Allow it to wash away all negative thought patterns and judgments.

Slowly, the liquid flows into your neck and shoulders, smoothing away knots and releasing burdens that you hold. Permit the liquid to flow into your heart center, washing away grief, anger, depression, and sadness...

Slowly, the liquid then flows into your upper back, relaxing your body so it sinks even more heavily into the surface that supports it. Let the warm, blue liquid drain down into your arms and flow into your hands and then into each finger. Feel the warmth and energy... and when you are ready, allow the liquid to flow out of your fingers, taking with it anything that you are ready and willing to let go of.

As the last of the blue liquid drains away, it leaves behind a body that is now transparent and weightless ... a body that is in a perfect place to heal, to integrate, and to balance.

When you are ready, stretch and move in ways that come natural to you. When your eyes open, you will feel refreshed.

Author's note: Lynne Greene has been a student of Kripalu Yoga since 1997. In 2000, she graduated from the AtmaYoga teacher training, founded by Christopher Ken Baxter. After working in the medical field for 15 years, she honors the way yoga addresses the mind, body connection. Lynne completed Shiva Rea's vinyasa yoga training in 2003 and enjoys putting yoga flows or vinyasas together to help create releases. She also loves working with creative visualization. Lynne is a daily practitioner of mindfulness meditation. Contact Lynne at Simply Yoga, 860-749-7257, or e-mail lynyog@aol.com.

Cruising... Magical Motorcycle Rider

Guided Imagery

Time: 15 minutes

Summary: This healing imagery is focused on releasing mental tension as well as physical pain. Troubles are left behind during an exhilarating motorcycle ride.

O O O

Let's take time to relax and find relief from your troubles and worries... relief from your aches and pain, a chance to heal and recover energy.

Gently close your eyes, and let them be still... Allow yourself to settle into your mat or chair... Take some time to move around a bit and make any changes that may help you be more comfortable... as this time is just for you.

Now bring your attention to my voice... and as you do, begin to let go of the cares of your day... allowing your troubles to dissolve for now... so you can feel relief.

Slowly, bring your attention to your breath and let it sink into its own natural, steady, effortless rhythm... Simply watching and feeling your breath... and your breath begins to soothe you... breathing easily... breathing freely... breathing evenly.

Now take in a deep, slow breath, comfortably filling your lungs... holding it for a moment... then letting go completely... Take in another slow, even breath... Hold it a moment... then let your breath out, let it release.

Fill up with soothing air... and let go completely as you breathe out... feeling the flow of breath throughout your body... just allowing your breath to connect inwardly... and whenever your thoughts drift away, simply bring your attention back to your breath... allowing as much of the tension, tightness, and pain as you can to flow out with your breath.

Now you begin to notice a warm, soothing wave of relaxation making its way from the top of your head all the way down to the tips of your toes ... that's right, slow and easy ... this warm flowing wave moves through your body, gathering up tension so it can be sent out through your feet, deep into the earth where it can be reused in another form.

Your breathing is becoming effortless and natural, and it has a way of slowing you down ... so all the negative feelings can be washed away ... so you can heal.

You let your scalp soften ... and the softness flows around your forehead ... and along your eyes ... down your cheeks and nose ... and across your mouth, unclenching your teeth so your jaw can relax ... letting go of tension and pain ... and you let go even more as the warmth flows down your neck and around your shoulders, taking the tightness with it as it continues down through your arms ... Now the tension is flowing right out your fingertips and away from you ... Imagine some of your tense, painful feelings melting away from you ... Imagine some of your tense, painful feelings melting right out your fingertips.

You feel the relaxation spreading to your chest and upper back ... and down into your belly ... comforting the rawness ... bringing relief.

Now imagine this wave of comfort moving gently down your back and then surrounding your hips and thighs ... bringing comfort ... Feel the tension begin to leave now as warmth blankets your knees, wrapping them in comfort ... surrounding and protecting your ankles and feet, right down to the tips of your toes. Allow the tension to drain from your body, letting it go away from you as it leaves through your feet.

You may have noticed that each time you breathe in, you feel more at ease, and each time you breathe out, you let go of tension and tightness ... unwinding and letting go.

Now imagine getting on a magical motorcycle ... it's your favorite make and model ... just the way you like it ... Notice its color ... its size ... the feel of it ... and how it smells ... This motorcycle was made just for you and it's all yours ... It fits you perfectly and you settle onto it.

It's your favorite kind of day and now it's time for a cruise ... You start the motor and your motorcycle springs to life. You hear its sound ... its power ... and you're off riding down the road, getting away from it all.

As you ride along, you feel the breeze and you are completely comfortable, cruising along ... watching the scenery go by and it brings a sense of freedom ... pure enjoyment ... of getting away from it all.

The motor is strong and steady, and you're cruising at just the right speed and you feel one with it all ... The scenery is beautiful, and you take it all in ... noticing the type of road you're on ... noticing your surroundings ... the colors ... the smells ... the sounds.

As you ride along, your mind begins to clear, and you gather your thoughts and go inside yourself to a place that feels wonderful ... where your own wisdom can come through ... as you ride on and on and on.

Pause.

And now, you come to a place where you can rest, perhaps get something to eat or drink ... It's a place where you can leave all your troubles behind and lighten your load ... and so you take some time to clear yourself out ... to let go.

Pause.

Now you get back on your bike, leaving your worries behind, and you ride again ... It's almost as if you are flying. The breeze blows right through you, cleaning out all the unwanted stuff so that when you come back, you'll feel fresher ... and lighter ... and better.

And now it's time to ride back ... Your attention returns to your breath, and your breathing is free. You feel refreshed and rested ... Whenever you are ready, you may stretch and open your eyes.

Author's Note: This visualization is dedicated to Rick Gilbert, a former coworker. Rick was in severe pain from the cancer that had invaded his bones. He was desperate for relief; however, he did not want to take too many drugs. One day I offered to customize a guided visualization for him and asked him what he enjoyed and wished he could do. He thought for a moment and replied that he would enjoy riding a motorcycle. I wrote and recorded Cruising for him and he listened to it often. Rick said that it reduced his pain, and his wife, Gail, added that it seemed to be the only thing that truly helped him relax. May he rest in peace.

Intuition Time

Guided Imagery

Time: 8 minutes

Summary: Age-old intuitive understanding and insights are revealed through an item of modern technology — the telephone. Have some paper and a pen handy to record whatever might be revealed.

Close your eyes and allow your entire body to relax comfortably ... settling yourself into whatever you are sitting or lying on. This is a time for you to let go of stress and strain, to enjoy your imagination through guided imagery.

Be still for a few moments and let go of muscular tightness and tension ... Start at your feet and work your way up your body, releasing tension as you go. Feel your body softening into the comfort of relaxation ... letting go of muscular tension ... Breathe in a way that is slow, smooth and deep ... taking time to breathe all the way in ... and all the way out ... slowly breathing in ... and out ... in ... and out ... relaxing further into the steady rhythm of your breath ... When your mind wanders, simply bring your attention to the steady stream of your breath ... sending any discomfort or tension out with your breath.

Imagine yourself nestled comfortably in an easy chair ... Sinking down even more comfortably ... let out an audible sigh ... Go ahead ... take a deep satisfying breath in ... and sigh it out.

Finally, you have some time to yourself to sort and sift through what's been happening lately ... so take a little time to consider what you've been doing ... how you've been feeling ... and what you've been thinking ... reviewing how things have been going.

As you ponder ... reflect on what's been running smoothly ... reviewing your relationships ... activities ... involvements ... health ... and anything else that has been prominent in your life ... considering all the areas in your life that are going well for you ... Let your mind run free to easily bring to mind all those things that are going well.

Pause.

Now it's time to begin to consider whatever has been puzzling you... That's right... explore in your mind's eye those things that have you stumped... once again, let your mind roam around and touch on those things... those relationships... those activities that you haven't had time to figure out and understand... or anything that has been troubling you for some time now.

Pause.

Using your mind's eye, imagine a telephone before you. It can be either modern or old-fashioned. What is it like?... As it becomes more real, you realize it's made so you can send and receive messages in a special way.

All of a sudden the phone rings... and it startles you for a second... You wonder who it could be... It rings a few more times, and you finally pick it up to see who it is.

The voice on the other end sounds familiar... however, you can't quite place it at first... Slowly, it dawns on you that it's someone who knows you well... and understands your heart of hearts... It's someone who takes your highest good seriously... Your heart lifts.

You realize that what has been puzzling you is understood perfectly by the caller... You ask for a fresh perspective to increase your understanding... knowing that if you'll just stop and listen for a while, the insights revealed will shed new light for you and help you on your way.

Pause.

It's time to say goodbye now... but before you do, promise to keep in touch with one another. All you have to do is reach out. Say your goodbyes... just for now.

It's time now for you to make a call. You can call anyone, anywhere... someone you know, someone you knew in the past, or someone you've always wanted to talk with. Go ahead, use the phone, make a connection, and begin communicating with your whole self.

When you're ready, stretch, open your eyes, and write down whatever you've learned.

Author's note: This exercise is dedicated to my brother, whose nickname was Tommy Telephone. On three occasions since his passing, the telephone has mysteriously rung a single time while I was focusing on him and asking him to stay in touch with me. Each time there has been nothing on Caller ID.

Heart Opening
Guided Imagery Meditations

As Patanjali says in the Yoga Sutras,
"The mind becomes clear and serene
when the qualities of the heart are cultivated:
friendliness toward the joyful, compassion toward the suffering,
happiness toward the pure, and impartiality toward the impure."
Yoga Sutras 1.33

The following mind-body practices will show you the way of safely and sweetly opening your heart.

Light a Candle
Meditation on the Universal Light (20 minutes)
Meta Meditation on Loving-Kindness (10 minutes or longer)
Awakening Compassion with Tonglen (15 minutes or longer)
Gratitude and Abundance (15 to 20 minutes)
Joy, Joy, Joy (10 to 15 minutes)

Light a Candle

Healing Practice

Summary: Light a candle as a help to remembering special people and circumstances.

Choose a candle and holder that is inspiring to you in some way. For this practice, I recommend a tea light and a lovely holder. A tea light burns for three to four hours and extinguishes itself.

Place the candle somewhere that you see and pass by often. A dining room or kitchen table works well. Be sure it is safe and away from anything it could catch on fire.

Light it with a blessing and the intention to help you remember special people and situations. Use your imagination. You may want to remember someone who is sick, going through difficult times, or making decisions. You may want to remember celebrations, such as birthdays, anniversaries, and other special occasions; people you love; or any person, event, or idea you want to keep on your mind.

Each time you see the light, your memory will be triggered. When this happens, recall whatever it is and if you like, say a prayer.

Consider telling people that you have lit a candle for them. In my experience, they are very appreciative.

Catholic churches are likely to have a candle altar. Anyone is welcome to light one for a minimal donation.

Authors note: As a child, I often lit a candle at church. It always felt powerful and healing to me. Throughout my life, my Mom would "light a big one" whenever I was being challenged or had to make a decision. Once again, it was comforting to know a light was burning on my behalf. One day it dawned on me that I could create a candle altar of my own in my home. Soon I realized how it served as a wonderful reminder for me to keep others in my heart and prayers.

Meditation on the Universal Light

Guided Imagery and Gazing Meditation

Contributed by Nischala Joy Devi

Time: 20 minutes

Summary: This wonderful meditation combines several techniques. As it progresses, it allows the benefits of your practice to spread out into the world. The method can be incorporated in many other meditations.

Place a candle on a table so that the flame is at eye level and two to three feet away.

Take a comfortable seated position with your spine erect, not leaning forward or backward or to the side. Close your eyes partially or fully. Begin to observe your body relaxing and letting go... Take in a few deep breaths and let them out very slowly... Allow your breath to return to normal... Observe it as it slowly flows in and out of your nostrils, easily without hesitation or strain.

Slowly open your eyes and gaze at a candle flame. Observe your breath... On each inhalation, begin to draw that light into your heart.

Continue to draw the light into your heart until you see one continuous flow from the candle to your heart.

As the light in your heart becomes brighter, allow your eyes to close and focus within.

Continue, with each inhalation, to see the flame in your heart brighten... On each exhalation, allow that same light to go out to the world as love.

On each inhalation, the light brightens... On each exhalation; send the light out to the world as love.

Three-minute pause.

Allow the love and light to grow and become the same size as your heart.

One-minute pause.

Allow the love and light to grow and become the same size as your entire physical body.

One-minute pause.

Allow the love and light to grow until it forms a body of light surrounding your physical body.

One-minute pause.

Allow the love and light to grow until it fills the entire room with love and light.

One-minute pause.

Allow the love and light to expand to all your family and friends, wherever they might be.

One-minute pause.

Allow the love and light to expand and embrace all the people, animals, plants, and minerals in this country.

One-minute pause.

Continue to expand to the north, south, east, and west, allowing the love and light to grow until it places a gentle covering of love and light around the entire earth and all her people, animals, plants, and minerals.

One-minute pause.

Expand this love and light into the far reaches of the universe and allow it to rest there.

Five-minute pause.

Slowly and gently, begin to bring your awareness back to the light in your own heart, the never-ending source of the love and light. Notice that, no matter how much you give out, the initial light is not diminished. Just as you can light a candle from an already-lit candle without the first candle losing any of its light, there is an abundant supply.

Allow your inhalation to deepen.

Feel yourself returning to your body.

Slowly allow your eyes to open slightly. Behold the first rays of light coming in. Allow the light from the outside to meet the light from within.

Continue to slowly open the eyes and allow the light from within to shine out into the world, wishing peace and love.

Author's note: This script was contributed by Nischala Joy Devi from her *Dynamic Stillness* CD. *Dynamic Stillness* is available from Abundant Well-Being, P.O. Box 346, Fairfax, CA 94978-0346, 888-543-8689 and at www.abundantwellbeing.com. Or write to nd@abundantwellbeing.com.

Nischala Joy Devi is a masterful, compassionate teacher and healer, who is highly respected and sought after as an international speaker and lecturer on yoga and its subtle uses in spiritual growth and healing. During her 18 years as a monk, she began discovering how to blend traditional western medicine with yoga and meditation. She then offered her expertise in developing the yoga portion of the Dr. Dean Ornish Program for Reversing Heart Disease, where she subsequently served for seven years as Director of Stress Management. She also cofounded the award-winning Commonweal Cancer Help Program.

With her knowledge of yoga and her experience in assisting those with heart disease, she created Yoga of the Heart™, a training and certification program for yoga teachers designed to adapt yoga practices to the special needs of cardiac patients. Nischala also produced the "Abundant Well-Being Series" relaxation CDs to allow these yoga and stress-relieving techniques to reach more people. Her book *The Healing Path of Yoga* expresses these teachings.

Meta Meditation on Loving-Kindness

Meditation

Time: 10 minutes or longer

Summary: The blessings of loving-kindness, peace, and protection are the subjects of this ancient meditation.

Meta meditation can be practiced by oneself or in a group. If it is done in a group, the leader can begin by saying "This is an ancient meditation that dates back thousands of years to Buddha. Every day, millions of people practice this loving-kindness meditation. I will say a line out loud, and then you can repeat it silently to yourself." The leader says one line at a time and leaves time enough for the others to repeat it silently. The leader also reads the guidance in italics. Every now and then, it is nice to have the group repeat the phrases aloud. It is also a nice touch to play meditative music, preferably live, between the verses. A Native American wooden flute works beautifully.

For a personal practice, reflect and meditate on each verse, letting each line soak into your heart. Each line or verse can be repeated as often as desired. Feel free to change the qualities and virtues to suit your preferences. Meta meditation is powerful as a daily practice.

Begin to settle your mind and body by sitting in a meditation posture. Use your breath or whatever method works well for you to clear your mind and open your heart.

May I be well.

May I be happy and peaceful.

May I be free from all danger and suffering.

May I be filled with loving-kindness.

Bring to mind a loved one and hold him or her in your thoughts while saying…

May you be well.

May you be happy and peaceful.

May you be free from all danger and suffering.

May you be filled with loving-kindness.

Bring to mind an acquaintance, such as a coworker or neighbor, and hold him or her in your thoughts while saying...

May you be well.

May you be happy and peaceful.

May you be free from all danger and suffering.

May you be filled with loving-kindness.

Bring to mind someone with whom you feel some friction, perhaps someone who you have a conflict with and hold that person in your thoughts while saying...

May you be well.

May you be happy and peaceful.

May you be free from all danger and suffering.

May you be filled with loving-kindness.

Bring to mind an animal or a pet.

May you be well.

May you be happy and peaceful.

May you be free from all danger and suffering.

May you be filled with loving-kindness.

Finally...

May all beings be well.

May all beings be happy and peaceful.

May all beings be free from danger and suffering.

May all beings be filled with loving-kindness.

Awakening Compassion with Tonglen
The Meditation of Giving and Receiving

Time: 15 minutes or more when practiced as a formal meditation

Tonglen is an advanced and powerful meditation practice from the Tibetan Buddhist tradition, which awakens and expands compassion. In this practice of giving and receiving, we inhale as we visualize taking on the pain and suffering of others; as we exhale, we see ourselves giving others all our happiness, well being, and positive resources. Our compassionate nature is strengthened as we transmute the inhaled pain and suffering into an exhalation of peace and freedom from suffering.

At first, Tonglen seems counterintuitive because it is based on breathing in unwanted qualities, such as darkness or anger, and breathing out the opposite, such as lightness or calmness. Courage is needed in order to feel personally strong enough for this practice. Some do not want to take in suffering, while others do not feel ready or capable of giving out the positive. The power of this practice derives from its ability to draw forth an inner well of strength and compassion we may not know we possess.

Tonglen can be done for anyone who is sick, hurt, in trouble or suffering, whether you do or do not know the person. It can, and especially in the early stages should, be done for ourselves, breathing in our own suffering and breathing out relief for ourselves. Tonglen can be done formally as a meditation practice, or "on the spot." When confronted with a situation that evokes your compassionate nature, you can practice breathing in the pain that is right before you and then sending out whatever will help.

Practicing Tonglen can create a distinct sense of relief because it generates a spacious feeling, especially on the exhalation. It gives you something specific to do with unwanted feelings and transforms them favorably. Furthermore, it causes a change of perspective, increases compassion, dissolves feelings of isolation, and opens the heart. The best way to discover the helpfulness of Tonglen is to try the formal practice and see for your self.

Sit in a meditative position and take a few minutes to breathe, rest your mind, and open your heart. Begin your Tonglen practice using yourself as the giver and the receiver.

Breathe in heaviness and darkness and breathe out lightness and brightness, or breathe in the feeling of being stuck and trapped and breathe out freedom and spaciousness. Use your personal preferences in color, sounds, feelings, words, or symbols to represent the heaviness and lightness.

Your breath rate should be natural and unforced. Place equal emphasis on each aspect of breathing in and out the qualities, taking time with this until it feels in synch with your breath. Gradually enlarge the experience until you feel like you are breathing through the pores of your body.

Next, bring to mind a personal situation. This could be anything that involves pain, unwanted thoughts, or other genuine feelings. Instead of avoiding your personal suffering, focus on and receive it with your incoming breath so it can be transformed into a sense of relief with each exhalation.

Once again, enlarge it past your mind's thoughts and send it in and out through your pores. Choose something that works for you. For example, you could counteract the negativity by visualizing a glorious sunrise or beautiful flower or by exchanging it for a peaceful feeling.

After a minute or two, change your focus from the story behind the feelings to just the feelings. Continue breathing in the unwanted feelings and radiating the opposite, giving each aspect the same amount of time. When you seem connected to this phase, move forward to the next one.

When you feel strengthened in your ability to take in pain and send out relief for yourself, you are ready to practice Tonglen for the sake of others. To do so, bring someone you care about and wish to help into your awareness and begin taking their suffering into yourself, transforming it, and breathing out relief. Once more, start with the story line in mind and then shift that into just the feelings themselves. If you get stuck, notice your own genuine reaction, receive it, transform it, and send out the opposite.

Next, enlarge the taking in and sending out so that it encompasses all those who are in the same situation, that is anyone else who has the same suffering, confusion, or problem. Breathe in their pain and send out relief. In this phase you are practicing Tonglen for yourself as well as for all others. Practice going back and forth between yourself and others if it is natural, and allow the subject matter or issue to shift as it happens.

To finish, take a few minutes to rest your mind and notice your breath.

Author's note: For years, this practice scared me to the bone, and I didn't want anything to do with it. I felt that it was better to decrease my sense of suffering and fear instead of bringing it inward, so I avoided Tonglen. The day of my brother's funeral, I was totally gripped with sorrow, grief, and despair and had no idea of how to manage the intense feelings that were ripping and pounding through me. Dan Roche, a dear friend, gave me the following verse by Joe Zarantonello. It says "Ripening are the wounded — who breathe in all the pain and loss and who breathe out simply some sense of relief for themselves and for all fellow sufferers." In my desperation, I stopped resisting the grief and acknowledged the depth of my feelings, and then I remembered to let go and breathe it all out. Amazingly, I felt the intensity decrease and felt spontaneous relief. I discovered the power of this practice when I needed it the very most. The grief returns as I write this, and I breathe it in, embrace it, and breathe out relief. It is an ongoing process, and Tonglen is truly something that helps me in my healing.

More on Tonglen can be learned from the writings and recordings of Pema Chödrön and Sogyal Rinpoche. Special thanks to Laurie Moon for sharing her insights and ideas with me concerning Tonglen.

Gratitude and Abundance

Guided Meditation

Time: 15 to 25 minutes

Summary: This two-part guided meditation generates gratitude. Gratitude is a doorway for discovering abundance everywhere — in the mundane, the mysterious, the miserable, and the miraculous. Abundance stretches far beyond financial and material wealth into the realm of appreciation for everything from the small to the significant. When gratitude and abundance are paired, a new, expansive perspective is discovered.

As the group leader, you can modify this exercise to meet your goals by including all the prompts, selecting appropriate ones for the group, or creating your own. The two parts can be separated into two experiences or combined as they are written.

This exercise can be done either in a meditative state or as a writing exercise. If it is done in writing, provide paper and pens, explain the purpose of the exercise, and create a positive atmosphere by spending some time with the centering exercise provided or one of your own. If done as a meditation, the experience will be even more powerful if time is provided at the end for people to write about their experiences.

Centering
Take some time to go inside yourself to settle your body, mind, and heart. Feel free to use whatever method works best for you ... focusing on your breath, a mantra, or stretching your body mindfully ... In your own way, remind yourself how being tenderhearted with yourself enriches all your relationships and circumstances.

The Attitude of Gratitude
Being grateful on a regular basis is a wonderful outlook on life. No matter what, there is always someone or something to appreciate. Gratitude is the foundation for many things ... It softens the heart ... generates generosity ... brings showers of grace ... satisfaction ... and serves as a foundation for abundance.

Today you'll be reflecting on different dimensions of your life with the attitude of gratitude. You will receive suggestions for recognizing what you are thankful for. I'll give you a prompt and you'll silently repeat and complete the statement "I am thankful for..."

Let's begin with simply saying, "I am thankful for..." completing the sentence for yourself. Do this over and over again, at your own pace, and notice what comes up.

Pause.

Now it's time to direct your attention to special areas of appreciation...so, just like you've been doing, complete the statement "I am thankful for..." except this time, focus on the material things you're grateful for.

Pause.

This time, focus on all the people you appreciate. "I am thankful for..."

Pause.

Now, call to mind the present circumstances that you are grateful for...being thankful for what's pleasing and desirable in your life.

Pause.

And now, the undesirable circumstances, from the perspective of gratitude and with faith in the lessons it has for you.

Pause.

Now, remember various circumstances from the past that you are grateful for...Start with desirable circumstances.

Pause.

And now, the undesirable circumstances from the past.

Pause.

Complete the statement "I am thankful for..." and reflect on personal qualities you have...and those you admire.

Pause.

Finally, let your mind roam to whatever else you appreciate.

Pause.

Notice what you are feeling in this moment...Explore what's happening in your heart area...and in your mind...and within yourself.

Pause.

Either conclude the experience or continue on as follows.

Abundance and Prosperity
Return to your breath or your way of centering.

Pause.

Bring to mind your dreams and desires ... either allow them to bubble up from inside or consciously choose whatever you would like to have more of in your life. This could be in any area that is meaningful to you.

Pause.

Visualize your dreams and desires coming to fruition ... and being complete. What will it be like when your wishes come true? ... What will it feel like?

Pause.

Acknowledge that abundance is all around and there is more than enough for you, in fact, there is enough for everyone ... Believe in your dreams ... and be ready to recognize opportunities as you put effort into your dreams and desires.

Pause.

To help yourself move along, let your dreams go ... release them ... so they can start manifesting in your life ... It doesn't help to try and control what and how and when things happen ... It does help to actively plant the seeds ... cultivate your resources ... and act on opportunities that are in accord with your dreams for abundance.

Pause.

It's time for this experience to come to a close and for you to make the transition back ... spend a few more minutes reflecting on your experience, and when you're ready, return your attention to the here and now and stretch.

Joy, Joy, Joy

Guided Meditation

Time: 10 to 15 minutes

Summary: Feeling joyful is always welcome. This meditation will connect you with the inner joy that is yours.

Depending upon your needs, other qualities, such as contentment, courage, and peace can be substituted for joy.

Take some time to go inside yourself to settle your body, mind, and heart. Feel free to use whatever method works best for you. You may want to focus on your breath, on a mantra, or on stretching your body mindfully... In your own way, remind yourself how being tenderhearted with yourself enriches all your relationships and circumstances.

Pause.

Bring your attention to your breathing and follow its natural course... breathing in ... breathing out... breathing in ... breathing out.

Shift your attention to your heart space... the place that is deep inside your heart center... and allow your attention to rest right inside your heart.

Continue breathing in a way that feels as if it's your heart that is breathing... feeling how the air stream flows in and out from your heart.

Now it's time to make more room in your heart for joy... not only for fleeting feelings of joy, but for the significant and substantial joy that is your true nature.

Call to mind a memory of a joyful occasion in your life... from a time in your distant past, or from recent times... just so it's a time that brings a smile and a feeling of happiness and delight.

For instance, remember a time you laughed so hard you cried... or a place where you feel totally at home... doing something that is pleasurable... If you prefer, you could recall the look of joy on someone else's face... seeing joy beam from their eyes... and from their heart... and connecting with your heart.

Relive the joy right now... noticing how it feels inside you... what it feels like in your heart... around your belly... in your head... And now, make room so the feeling of joyfulness can spread and expand.

Stay with the feelings of joy and delight and let go of the story line... allow the memories to fade... and allow the feeling of happiness to remain.

Breathe into the center of the happiness and joy and with each breath... feel the joyfulness expand... as if you are stoking a fire... while sparks of light radiate all around... illuminating your body, mind, and heart with joy.

Anchor this experience inside yourself by making a small gesture. For example, you could gently touch your thumb and pinky finger together, creating a touchstone enabling you to return to this wellspring of joyfulness whenever you want... Imagine planting the feeling inside this gesture so you will be able to access this internal source of joy whenever you would like... by simply quieting yourself for a moment and repeating the gesture. The more you practice this whole sequence, the better it will work and the more joy and abundance you will experience.

When you are ready, stretch and acknowledge the joy and pleasure of physical movement... the joy of your breath... and the joy of being alive.

Chakras: Centers of
Subtle Energy

Each of us has seven subtle energy centers that influence our health and well-being and involve every system of the body. The energy of the chakras is often described as the most important indicator of a person's well-being. They guide the developmental stages of our body, mind, and emotions and awaken our evolutionary potential as spiritual beings. They are said to house the guiding intelligence of the universal energy of life. Yogis refer to this life force as prana; the Chinese masters call it chi; and the Japanese practitioners name it ki. The chakras were first referenced in one of the oldest of the yogic texts, known as the Atharva Veda, probably compiled in the third millennium B.C.E. The Upanishads and the Yoga Sutras of Patanjali also refer to the chakras. Many medical, mental health, spiritual, and mind-body professionals and practitioners now seek to understand and apply the ancient knowledge of the chakras within their field of expertise.

Traditionally, the seven primary chakras are described as spinning wheels of subtle energy that span from the base of the spine to the crown of the head. Each of the seven chakras is associated with and has an influence on, physical locations in the body as well as on adjacent muscles, organs, glands, and nerves. Furthermore, each is related to stages of psychological growth and human development and has lessons that are integral to our soul's journey. Because they are energetic rather than physical structures, they are not considered to be a physical part of our biology. In contemporary language, they are described as psycho-energetic or psycho-spiritual centers located in the subtle body. In other words, like magnetism existing within an iron magnet or electricity within a light bulb, they exist within the body without having a physical presence. Each of the chakras is also associated with a rainbow color, element, and sounds. Their influence is present in every moment of life and in every cell of the body. Refer to the chakra chart for detailed information.

The current of chakra energy flow moves both vertically and horizontally. When the chakras are unbalanced by either a surplus or shortage of energy, the result is physical, mental, emotional, or spiritual difficulties. The same source of wisdom that has recognized and worked with the chakras for eons has provided a wide range of techniques to open, align, and activate the chakras.

The guided meditations and affirmations presented here incorporate these wisdom teachings. Locations, colors, lessons and sounds associated with balancing the chakras are provided in a safe and balanced manner. Sitting in a meditation posture is more effective than lying down for working with the chakras because the physical alignment encourages and amplifies the flow of energy. Although there are many yoga poses and other activities that can be of help, I have selected one main asana for each chakra to help get you started. Regular practice of the meditations and postures will have a positive effect on your overall well-being: physically, mentally, energetically, and spiritually.

Energy Flow (12 to 15 minutes)

The Chakra Rainbow (12 to 15 minutes)

Chakra Affirmations (10 minutes)

Root Chakra: Security and Safety (15 minutes)

Sacral Chakra: Pleasure and Creativity (15 minutes)

Solar Plexus Chakra: Personal Confidence, and Self-esteem (15 minutes)

Heart Chakra: Love, Peace of Heart, and Compassion (15 minutes)

Throat Chakra: Communication and Expression (15 minutes)

Third Eye Chakra: Insight and Intuition (15 minutes)

Crown Chakra: Cosmic Consciousness (15 minutes)

Sources for the Chakra Chart on the following pages include Anodea Judith, Jeff Migdow, Barbara Pritchard, and Rosalyn Bruyere.

Chakra Chart	1 Root Muladhara	2 Sacral Svadhisthana	3 Solar Plexus Manipura
Location	Base of Spine, Legs	Pelvis, Low back, Abdomen	Solar Plexus
Endocrine System	Adrenals	Ovaries, Testis	Pancreas, Adrenals
Element	Earth	Water	Fire
Primary Color	Red	Orange	Yellow
Balancing Color	Green	Blue	Violet
Lesson	Self-preservation	Self-gratification	Self-definition
Rights and Responsibilities	To have, to be here	To feel, to want, to create	To act
Balanced Chakra Energy	Feels safe and secure Physically healthy Good body image Right livelihood Prosperous Lives in here and now Able to be still	Emotional intelligence Graceful movement Able to change Can nurture self and others Healthy boundaries Feels pain and pleasure Sensual satisfaction	Self-confident Good self-esteem Right action Healthy boundaries Takes responsibility Disciplined Creative Sense of belonging
Challenges	Fear	Guilt	Shame
Excessive Chakra Energy	Sluggishness Heaviness Monotony Hoarding Materialistic Greedy Workaholic	Too sensitive Obsessive Poor boundaries Emotional dependency Excessive mood swings Instability Sensual/sexual addictions	Domineering Blaming Aggressive Flighty Hyperactive Competitive
Deficient Chakra Energy	Fear, Anxiety Lacks discipline Spacey Difficulty manifesting Resists structure	Emotional numbness Fear of pleasure Fear of change Lacking passion Bored, Frigid, Impotent	Weak will Poor self-esteem Submissive Fearful Lacking energy
Musical Note	C Drum	D Brass	E Sax
Bija Mantra to Increase & Attract	Lam as in "Lum"	Vam as in "Vum"	Ram "Rum" with rolling R
Vowel Sounds to Release & Send	O as in "toe"	OO as in "two"	Ah as in "awe"
Breathing Practices	Dirgha breath complete breath	Dirgha breath complete breath	Kapalabhati breath of fire
Yoga Postures	Foot and leg stretches Seated, lying and standing poses Core lift Forward fold Locust Child Lie face down or up	Cobra Cat stretches Seated hip openers Core lift Bound angle Standing hip circles and stretches Eagle or cow legs	Core lift Abdominal exercises Sun salute Warrior I, Twists Boat / Cobra Restorative backbends Spinal twist Forward fold
Other Healing Activities	Walk, Hike Play Garden Right eating & sleeping Work with hands Eat proteins & vegetables	Drink water Bathe, Swim Increase flexibility Dance Enjoy senses Experience emotions Drink water & juice	Get moving Break attachments Take risks Release anger Nurture self, Laugh Balance light & dark Eat whole grains

4 Heart Anahata	5 Throat Vissudha	6 Third Eye Ajna	7 Crown Sahasrara
Heart, Lungs, Arms	Throat, Ears, Mouth, Hands	Brow, Between Eyebrows	Top of Head
Thymus	Thyroid	Pineal, Pituitary	Beyond the body
Air	Ether / Sound	Mind / Light	Beyond elements
Green	Blue	Indigo	Violet / White
Red	Orange	Yellow (deep)	Yellow (pale)
Self-acceptance	Self-expression	Self-reflection	Self-knowledge
To love & be loved	To create, speak & be heard	To see, to witness	To know
Loving, Caring Compassionate Accepting Loves self & others Peaceful, Content Centered Trusting Non-judgmental	Full, resonant voice Communicates clearly with others Good self-expression Good listener Truthful Creative expression	Strong intuition Insightful Imaginative Good memory Good dream recall Has guiding vision for life Able to watch & witness Can see the big picture	Spiritually connected Wisdom & mastery Intelligence Presence Able to question Able to assimilate & analyze information Open mind
Grief	Deceit	Illusion	Attachment
Codependent (too much focus on others) Poor boundaries Jealous Being a martyr Being a pleaser	Excessive talking Unable to listen Over-extended Gossiping, Too loud Unable to keep secrets Forcing creative expression	Trouble concentrating Headaches Intrusive memories Excessive fantasizing Nightmares Obsessions Delusions	Too intellectual Spiritual addiction Confusion Detached from spirit Dissasociated from body Living "in your head"
Antisocial Withdrawn Critical, Intolerant Lonely, Isolated Lacking empathy	Fear of speaking Poor rhythm Weak voice Excessive shyness Denies creativity	Insensitive, Denial Poor memory Poor vision Can't see patterns Unimaginative, Inflexible	Trouble learning Spiritual uncertainty Limited beliefs Materialistic Apathy, Closed mind
F Violin	G Flute	A Crystal bowl	B Voice
Yam as in "Yum"	Ham as in "Hum"	Om	Beyond sound
A as in "play"	EE as in "speak"	Mmmm	ING as in wing or silence
Nadi Shodhana alternate nostril	Ujjayi breath ocean breath	Breath of Fire alternate nostril	Nadi Shodhana alternate nostril
Chest & shoulder openers Backbends to increase energy Fish, Cobra Bridge Forward bends to decrease energy	Neck & shoulder stretches Bridge Shoulder stand Fish (supported) Fish Camel	Eye exercises Gazing Close eyes Spinal twist Yoga Mudra	Inversions Headstand Yoga Mudra Balance poses
Breathwork Practice acceptance of self & others Forgiveness Gratitude, love Eat vegetables	Chanting, Singing Being silent Listen to or create music Be creative, Journal Eat fruits	Meditate Enjoy & create beauty Create visual art Visual stimulation Abstain from food Breathe	Meditate, Pray Enjoy creativity Experience beauty Use your brainpower Learn Define beliefs & values Abstain from food Breathe

Energy Flow

Guided Imagery

Time: 12 to 15 minutes

Summary: Energy flows like a river in this guided imagery exercise. Sitting in a meditation posture is more effective than lying down for working with the chakras because the physical alignment encourages and amplifies the flow of energy.

Each of us has internal currents of energy within that flow like rivers. This energy is what gives us life and activates us physically, mentally, emotionally and spiritually. It influences everything from the concrete to the abstract. Our flesh and bones are activated into life by this energy source; it gives us inspiration to accomplish our meaningful ambitions. Primarily, these rivers of energy travel from the base of the spine through the top of the head, moving up and down, in and out, forward and back. Furthermore, there are many other tributaries that extend throughout the rest of our being.

When this energy is open, flowing, and balanced, we're able to express our full potential and interact with the outside world. It enables us to easily receive information, love, and resources from outside of us. We're also able to manifest our dreams and life purpose, liberate our awareness and actions, and free up energy to take action. It's important for this energy to flow in a balanced, continuous way. Too often however, areas of energy become overly stimulated and excessive, or energy bogs down, gets blocked, or leaky.

The purpose of this guided imagery is to balance these rivers and currents of energy in a wholesome way. So in your own manner, set an intention to balance and align your energy flow so it serves the greater good for yourself… others… and in the world.

In your own way, become aware of a constant source of energy and power that is plentiful… and readily available to you as well as to all others… There are many ways of experiencing the energy as it flows, and you can use your senses to help experience it… Perhaps you can see it, feel it, or hear it … It may have a color, a shape or a sound … It may possibly sparkle … it may glow … How does the presence of energy occur to you?

Imagine tapping into this energy supply right now. Feel it moving and flowing now.

Let's refine and focus on this energy more attentively by experiencing it as a fountain that flows from below your feet … and into your legs … and into the base of your spine … moving upward to the top of your head and beyond … a constant fountain of energy that flows, and moves and is alive … actively flowing through the core of your body from the base to the top … Imagine this energy lighting up your awareness … increasing your freedom … and liberating you.

Pause.

And now, imagine this energy as it showers down like a waterfall. It originates above you and pours down through the crown of your head, down throughout the core of your body, and back to the earth … Experience streams of energy running downward through you, boosting and enlivening your thoughts, dreams, and aspirations into reality … and clearly imagine your dreams taking shape in the world.

Pause.

So now, this energy flows evenly and fluidly … gracefully moving up and down … up and down the central core that spans from the top of your head to the base of your spine and back to the crown of your head … It can even extend from the earth, through you, into the sky and back down again.

Allow this energy to continually flow … automatically … fluidly … and elegantly … whether or not you are paying direct attention to it.

Now it's time to experience this flow of energy in a new way … This river of energy influences your incoming and outgoing interactions … so hold your attention on the whole length of your spine, from its base to the top … Allow a wellspring of energy to radiate constantly through the length of your spine … and feel it start to move in and out … forward and back … and sideways … Imagine a constant, abundant supply of energy radiating out from your core … energy shining out through the front … out the back … to the sides … and all around … making it possible for you to express your self in your life … including your work … touching your relationships … and the world you live in … as this energy moves along the length of your spine, radiating outward in all directions.

And now, this energy returns to you, moving from the outside to the inside...replenishing your energy...receiving it in its many forms...in the form of information...thoughts...and love...all being returned to you...naturally flowing into you until it begins flowing in and out like a dance...evenly...smoothly...and effortlessly...continuing to flow, whether or not you are paying attention to it.

And somehow, energy currents are flowing in all directions...up and down...in and out...in unison, balancing and blending and harmonizing...cooling and calming where the energy is excessive and too strong...and activating and energizing where the energy is too weak or blocked.

Pause.

Part of you steps out of the way so this can happen naturally...and this part of you notices how it all happens.

This energy source is inside you and all around you...It is constant and supportive...and it guides you...balances you...and makes you feel whole and complete.

Pause.

It's time to reawaken to your surroundings...Listen to the sounds *(name some as they occur)*...Become aware of your breath...Feel the air on your skin...Feel your body, your physical presence...And when you are ready, stretch and open your eyes.

Author's note: Anodea Judith inspired this guided visualization. May her energy be abundant and a blessing to herself and to all others.

The Chakra Rainbow

When the rainbow appears in the clouds, I will see it, that I may remember the everlasting covenant between God and all living beings on earth.
                                                            Genesis 9:16

Guided Imagery

Time: 12 to 15 minutes

Summary: Balancing and aligning the chakras with the colors and meanings associated with them is the purpose of this guided imagery exercise. Be sure to review the chakra description and chart at the beginning of this chapter for further information.

Sitting upright is more effective than lying down for chakra meditation. The physical alignment encourages and amplifies the flow of energy.

Variation: Magnify the effects of this experience by placing your hands over each chakra as it is highlighted.

Close your eyes and take time to go inside yourself to settle your body, mind, and heart. Feel free to use whatever method works best for you. You might pay attention to your breath, stretch your body mindfully, repeat a sound, word, or phrase, or focus on an image…In your own way, remind yourself how being compassionate with yourself is balancing and nurturing and provides you with inner strength.

Pause.

We are going to focus on each of the seven major power centers, called chakras, one at a time…The purpose is to balance and align them in a healing and supportive way…This will be done by using their associated colors, which relate to the colors of the rainbow. They start with the color red at the base of the spine and move upward to the crown of the head and the color violet. Some people can "see" the colors with their mind's eye, while others can't. It doesn't really matter. If you can't "see" them, that's fine. Simply experience the chakra energy however it occurs to you. Some experience the chakras as light, heat, or coolness, or even a tingly feeling. Just go with whatever you get.

Bring your attention to the root chakra located at the base of the spine...The color associated with the root chakra is red...Visualize the color red...Perhaps call to mind something that is red, like a red flower...and imagine red surrounding the base of your spine...See the red color protecting and stabilizing you with safety and security...surrounding the base of your spine with the color red.

Move your attention upward to the sacral chakra located in the lower abdomen and pelvis...The color orange is associated with the sacral chakra...Visualize the color orange...Imagine it surrounding and enfolding the lower back, abdomen and pelvis...See the orange color balancing your feelings and emotions...and making it possible for your personal wants and needs to be satisfied in a healthy way...feeling orange pour throughout the sacral chakra.

Notice the color red around the base of the spine...and the color orange around your lower abdomen and pelvis.

Move your attention upward to the chakra located at the solar plexus. This is the area located between the naval and the heart...see the color yellow shining in and around the solar plexus...stoking your sense of self-esteem in a positive way...helping you feel confident...and act responsibly...surrounding the sacral chakra with the color yellow.

Notice red around the base of your spine...and orange around your lower abdomen and pelvis...and yellow radiating from the solar plexus.

Move your attention upward to your heart chakra...This encompasses your lungs and heart...In your own way, give it the color green...spring green...visualizing or feeling the color green surrounding and gently embracing your heart and lungs...soaking it with love and compassion...and the color green.

Notice the color red around the base of your spine...and the color orange around your lower abdomen and pelvis...and yellow radiating from the solar plexus...and green gently embracing your heart chakra...feeling the flow of movement and color from the base of your spine to your heart.

Move your attention upward to the throat chakra...this includes your neck, throat, mouth and ears...imagine the color blue, a sky blue, enfolding your throat...clearing the way for being capable of expressing yourself through your words and actions...Visualize the color blue comforting and clearing the throat chakra.

Once again, feel the movement of energy starting at the base of your spine and moving upward. Start with the color red around the base of your spine...and the color orange around your lower back, abdomen, and pelvis...and yellow radiating from your solar plexus...and green gently embracing your heart chakra...and now a clear blue around your throat.

Move your attention upward to the chakra located in the center of the brow, the third eye...The color associated with the third eye is indigo...Visualize indigo in the center of your forehead...sparking your intuition and imagination...with the color of indigo.

Draw your attention to the base of your spine and move upward. Start with red around the base of your spine...and orange around your lower abdomen and pelvis...and yellow radiating from your solar plexus...and green gently embracing your heart chakra...and a clear blue all around your throat...until there is an indigo light shining from the center of your forehead.

Move your attention upward to the crown chakra at the top of your head...there is a clear violet light associated with the crown chakra...see a clear violet light glowing at the top of your head...Feel a growing connection to your true Self...your higher Self...and see a beautifulviolet light emanating from the crown of your head...and extending upwards.

Pause.

And now, draw your attention down through the chakras...from the violet color at the crown of your head...to the indigo at the forehead...flowing down to the blue at your throat...and on to green radiating from your heart...descending to a yellow shining from your solar plexus...and downward to an orange streaming all around your sacral chakra...until it reaches the base of your spine which is red.

And back up again...red...orange...yellow...green...blue...indigo...and violet...allowing the stream of colors to flow up and down...clearing and energizing you from the base of your spine to the crown of the head and back down, circling through the chakras as they activate and balance...Feel the movement and the flow of the energy.

Perhaps there is a location or a color that is particularly attractive and appealing to you...If this is true for you now, go with that color or place...Trust that what is happening is for your greater good and go with it for a while.

Pause.

Let your body be like a rainbow of color that is supporting you and lighting your way...tenderly and lovingly...right now...doing its healing and balancing work...harmonizing the chakras in a way that supports you and your life purpose.

Focus your awareness along the entire column of chakras...aligned, balanced and glowing beautifully.

As you're ready, begin stretching, and when your eyes open, you'll feel alert and vibrant.

Chakra Affirmations

Affirmations

Time: 10 minutes

Summary: Affirmations are brief, constructive statements said in the present tense and repeated often to improve mental attitudes and to assist in making positive changes. These affirmations are based upon chakras, the seven subtle energy centers of the body.

Say the following affirmations, either silently or aloud.

Chakra One:

I am safe and sound, protected in my own personal sanctuary.

I am grounded and feel steady, strong, and stable.

I belong.

Chakra Two:

I have the right to feel my emotions.

My own creativity flows abundantly like a waterfall freely streaming.

I feel pleasure in healthy ways.

Chakra Three:

I am healthy and happy in body, mind, heart and soul, glowing like the rays of the sun.

My willpower serves the meaning and purpose of my life.

My life unfolds according to plan.

I am confident.

Chakra Four:

My heart is strong and sensitive.

My heart flows with compassion for myself and others.

Love gently and abundantly blows through my life like the breeze on a beautiful day.

Chakra Five:

I communicate my thoughts and feelings with crystal clarity.

I speak and hear the truth, sounding like an expressive melody.

I have the right to be heard.

Chakra Six:

My innate intelligence and insight is wise.

Wisdom guides me and lights up my intuition.

More and more, I trust my instincts.

Chakra Seven:

I am connected to the infinite life source.

I belong.

Recorded on *Wholesome Relaxation* CD by Julie Lusk with music by Tom Laskey. Available from Whole Person Associates at 800-247-6789 or on the Web at wholeperson.com.

Introduction to the
Seven Chakra Meditations

Each of the next seven meditations focuses on one chakra at a time. To develop a deeper understanding of each chakra and to bring it into balance, the name and location of each chakra is identified; its color is imagined; affirmations are used to highlight the basic rights and lessons associated with it; and its healing sounds are toned.

Feel free to either practice each meditation in its entirety or to focus on a portion of it. For example, focus on the location and color of a chakra during one meditation session; then on other occasions, concentrate on either its affirmations or its sounds. Always be alert to the internal changes that occur.

Before proceeding, please familiarize yourself with the chakra overview at the beginning of this chapter and review the information contained in the chakra chart. If you are leading others, be sure to give participants a synopsis of the chakras first, particularly the one being highlighted.

Root Chakra / Muladhara

Guided Imagery, Affirmations, and Healing Sound

Time: 15 minutes

Muladhara is pronounced MOOL-ah-dah-ra

Summary: The first chakra is the root chakra. It is located deep inside, at the base of the spine. It is related to the fundamental awareness associated with safety, security and survival. Feeling safe, being physically healthy, having a good body image, being able to live in the here and now, and having the ability to be still are signs of a balanced root chakra. Its color is predominantly red, and its sounds are Lam (pronounced Lum) and O (as in toe).

❁ ❁ ❁

Prepare yourself by sitting in an upright meditative position. Please make sure that your spine is straight. Close your eyes or keep them barely open.

Bring your attention to your breath and follow its pattern as you breathe in ... and out ... Allow your breath to become smooth ... and full ... breathing so that the inhalation and the exhalation are balanced.

Gradually, allow your exhalation to become longer than your inhalation ... Allowing this to happen is relaxing and centering.

Send your awareness to the area of your tailbone at the base of your spine. This is where the root chakra is located. Take a few moments to explore and experience the sensations felt at the base of your spine.

Pause.

Maintain your awareness at the base of your spine and return your attention to your breath ... so now you are maintaining your focus at the base of your spine as well as on your breathing ... If your mind wanders, simply bring your attention back to your breath and to the base of your spine ... If it's easier to maintain your awareness either on your breath or the base of your spine, choose one and allow your attention to settle there.

Pause.

Call to mind the color red. This is the color associated with the first chakra ... Sense the color in any way you wish. Imagine, perhaps, the red color of an apple ... or a flower ... or a car ... In your mind's eye, allow the redness to liquefy ... or become a red mist ... or transform into a red light ... and imagine it bathing and soaking and surrounding the base of your spine ... sensing a cleansing red liquid ... a glowing light ... or a healing red mist at the base of your spine.

Pause.

The root chakra represents your right and responsibility to be alive ... and your right to be here and have your needs met. ... Resolving and letting go of fear is healthy and one of the lessons of the first chakra.

To help you integrate these lessons into your being, repeat the following statements aloud or silently.

"I have the right to be here.". I belong

"I have the right to have my needs met."

Pause. Repeat the affirmations every so often during the pause.

Notice what happens as you say these statements to yourself.

How do you react to these basic rights?

"I release and let go of my fears."

Pause.

"I am safe.". Protected inside of my body (my own personal sanctuary)

Pause.

This next part involves the use of sound. The sound of the first chakra is Lam *(pronounced as lum with the lu held longer than the m)*. The sound of Lam will send a healing sound vibration to strengthen and balance your first chakra. First it will be said aloud, next it will be whispered, and finally it will be said silently. Each step will be repeated three times.

Now take a full breath in and repeat the sound of Lam out loud while exhaling ... Repeat the sound Lam over and over as you exhale, doing so for three breaths.

Breathe in ... Say Lam, Lam, Lam, Lam ... while breathing out.

Repeat two more times.

Pause.

Continue whispering Lam for three breaths.

Pause long enough for this to take place.

Continue saying Lam silently for three breaths.

Pause long enough for this to take place.

Now let the Lam sound echo on by itself.

Pause.

The sound oooooooo (as in toe) will continue to balance the first chakra and it will release and send the energy out to share.

This time, take a full breath and say a long ooooooooo out loud for three breaths.

Pause long enough for this to take place.

Continue whispering oooooooo for three breaths.

Pause long enough for this to take place.

Continue saying oooooooo silently for three breaths.

Pause long enough for this to take place.

Now, let the oooooooo sound echo on by itself.

Pause.

Now, take some time on your own to focus on the location, color, lessons (or sounds) of the root chakra ... (simply follow your own inclination)... You could focus on the sensations at the base of the spine... the color red ... your right and responsibility to be alive ... to release fear ... to feel safe ...(Perhaps; you would feel most at ease repeating Lam or oooooooo. Simply follow your own inclination for the next few minutes.)

Longer pause.

It's time to make the transition back ... Return your attention to your surroundings ... feeling whatever you are sitting on ... listening to the sounds in this space... and becoming more and more aware of your breath and your body ... When you are ready, stretch and open your eyes.

Sacral Chakra / Svadhisthana

Guided Imagery, Affirmations, and Healing Sound

Time: 15 minutes

Svadhisthana is pronounced SVAH-dees-tah-nah

Summary: The second chakra is the sacral chakra and is located deep within the lower abdomen and pelvis. It is associated with being able to feel, want and create in relation to personal and physical needs. With a balanced sacral chakra, you are emotionally intelligent, able to nurture your self and others, and have healthy boundaries. You are able to move gracefully, enjoy sensual satisfaction, and experience an array of emotions ranging from pain to pleasure. Its color is predominantly orange, and its sounds are Vam (pronounced Vum) and O (as is two).

Prepare yourself by sitting in an upright meditative position. Please make sure that your spine is straight. Close your eyes or keep them barely open.

Bring your attention to your breath and follow its pattern as you breathe in ... and out ... Allow your breath to become smooth ... and full ... breathing so that the inhalation and the exhalation are balanced.

Gradually, allow your exhalation to become longer than your inhalation ... Allowing this to happen is relaxing and centering.

Send your awareness to your naval center. This consists of the pelvic bowl and low back and goes deep inside your lower abdomen. Generally, it's an inch or two below your navel. This is where the sacral chakra is located. Take a few moments to explore and experience the sensations felt in your naval center ... the abdominal organs ... low back ... and pelvis.

Pause.

Maintain your awareness at the sacral chakra and return your attention to your breath ... so now you are keeping your focus on your pelvis and navel center as well as on your breathing ... If your mind wanders, simply bring your attention back to your breath and to the sacral charka ... If it's easier to maintain your awareness either on your breath or the sacral chakra, choose one ... and allow your attention to settle there.

Pause.

Call to mind the color orange … sensing the color in any way you wish. Perhaps, imagine the color of an orange … or an orange flower … or the orange color of a sunset… In your mind's eye, allow the orange image to become an orange liquid … a light … or a mist … and imagine it within and around your naval center … sensing a cleansing orange liquid, a glowing light, or an orange healing mist filling your pelvic bowl.

Pause.

The sacral chakra represents your right and responsibility to feel … your right to want … and the right to nurture yourself in response to your personal, human needs … Resolving and letting go of guilt is healthy and is one of the lessons of the sacral chakra.

To help you integrate these lessons into your being, repeat the following statements aloud or silently.

"I have the right to feel"

"I have the right to self satisfaction."

"I have the right to respond to my own needs."

Pause. Repeat the affirmations every so often during the pause.

Notice what happens as you say these statements to yourself.

How do you react to these basic rights?

Pause.

"I release and let go of guilt."

Pause.

"I feel pleasure in healthy ways."

Pause.

This next part involves the use of sound. The sound of the second chakra is Vam"*(pronounced as vum with the vu held longer than the m)*. The sound of Vam will send a healing sound vibration to strengthen and balance your second chakra. First it will be said out loud, next it will be whispered, and finally it will be said silently. Each step will be repeated three times.

Breathe in … Say Vam, Vam, Vam, Vam … while breathing out.

Repeat two more times.

Pause long enough for this to take place.

Continue whispering Vam for three breaths.

Pause long enough for this to take place.

Continue saying Vam silently for three breaths.

Pause long enough for this to take place.

Now let the Vam sound echo on by itself.

Pause.

The sound oooooooo (as in two) will continue to balance the second chakra and it will release and send the energy out to share.

This time, take a full breath and say a long ooooooooo out loud for three breaths.

Pause long enough for this to take place.

Continue whispering ooooooooo for three breaths.

Pause long enough for this to take place.

Continue saying ooooooooo silently for three breaths.

Pause long enough for this to take place.

Now, let the ooooooooo sound echo on by itself.

Pause.

Now, take some time on your own to focus on the location, color, lessons or sounds of the sacral chakra...simply follow your own inclination...You could focus on the sensations at your pelvis and navel center...the color orange...your right and responsibility to feel, to want, to create...to release guilt...to feel pleasure and creativity...Perhaps; you would feel most at ease repeating Vam or ooooooooo. Simply follow your own inclination for the next few minutes.

Longer pause.

It's time to make the transition back...Return your attention to your surroundings...feeling whatever you are sitting on...listening to the sounds in this space...and becoming more and more aware of your breath and your body...When you are ready, stretch and open your eyes.

Solar Plexus Chakra / Manipura

Knowledge of the whole body is obtained
through concentration and meditation on the navel center.

Yoga Sutra 3.30

Guided imagery, Affirmations, and Healing Sound

Time: 15 minutes

Manipura is pronounced MAH-nee-poor-ah

Summary: The third chakra is the solar plexus chakra, which is located between the naval and the heart. It is associated with accepting yourself, having good self-esteem and being personally powerful in the external world. Feeling self-confident, taking right action, being self-responsible and disciplined, and having a sense of belonging are signs of a balanced third chakra. Its color is predominantly yellow, and its sounds are Ram (pronounced Rum with a rolling r) and A (as in awe).

Prepare yourself by sitting in an upright meditative position. Please make sure that your spine is straight. Close your eyes or keep them barely open.

Bring your attention to your breath and follow its pattern as you breathe in...and out...Allow your breath to become smooth...and full...breathing so that the inhalation and the exhalation are balanced.

Gradually, allow your exhalation to become longer than your inhalation...Allowing this to happen is relaxing and centering.

Send your awareness to your solar plexus; it is located deep inside, between your navel and your heart. This is where the solar plexus chakra is located. Take a few moments to explore and experience the sensations felt in your solar plexus.

Pause.

Maintain your awareness at your solar plexus and bring your attention back to your breath...so now you are keeping your focus on your solar plexus as well as on your breathing...If your mind wanders, bring your attention back to your breath and to the solar plexus charka...If it's easier to maintain your awareness either on your breath or the solar plexus chakra, choose one...and allow your attention to settle there.

Pause.

Call to mind the color yellow ... sensing the color in any way you wish. Perhaps, imagine the color of a lemon ... a banana ... or a glowing sunflower ... In your mind's eye, allow the yellow image to transform into a yellow liquid ... light ... or mist ... and imagine it within and around your solar plexus ... sensing a cleansing yellow liquid ... a glowing yellow light ... or a healing mist in and around your solar plexus.

Pause.

The solar plexus chakra represents the life lesson that you have the right and responsibility to have inner strength ... You have the right to feel positive about yourself ... and you have the right to act with abundant energy ... Resolving and letting go of the shame of expressing and enjoying your own uniqueness and strength is healthy and a lesson of the third chakra.

To help you integrate these lessons into your being, repeat the following statements aloud or silently.

"I have the right to act."

"I have the right to feel positive about my true self."

Pause. Repeat the affirmations every so often during each pause.

Notice what happens as you say these statements to yourself.

How do you react to these basic rights?

Pause.

"I release and let go of shame."

Pause.

"I am my true self."

Pause.

This next part involves the use of sound. The sound of the third chakra is Ram *(pronounced as Rum with the ru held longer than the m. Roll the R by placing the tip of the tongue at the roof of your mouth).* The sound of Ram will send a healing sound vibration to strengthen and balance your third chakra. First it will be said out loud; next it will be whispered; and finally it will be said silently. Each step will be repeated three times.

Now take a full breath in and repeat the sound of Ram out loud while exhaling ... Repeat the sound Ram over and over as you exhale, doing so for three breaths.

Breathe in ... say Ram, Ram, Ram, Ram ... while breathing out.

Repeat two more times.

Pause.

Continue whispering Ram for three breaths.

Pause long enough for this to take place.

Continue saying Ram silently for three breaths.

Pause long enough for this to take place.

Now let the Ram sound echo on by itself.

Pause.

The sound aaaahhh (as in awe) will continue to balance the third chakra and it will release and send the energy out to share.

Take a full breath and say a long aaaahhh out loud for three breaths.

Pause long enough for this to take place.

Continue whispering aaaahhh for three breaths.

Pause long enough for this to take place.

Continue saying aaaahhh silently for three breaths.

Pause long enough for this to take place.

Now, let the aaaahhh sound echo on by itself.

Pause.

Now, take some time on your own to focus on the location, color, lessons, or sounds of the solar plexus chakra ... simply follow your own inclination ... You could focus on the sensations at your solar plexus ... the color yellow ... or your right and responsibility to be true to your self ... to release shame ... and to take action ... Perhaps you would feel most at ease repeating Ram or aaaaahhhh. Simply follow your own inclination for the next few minutes.

Longer pause.

It's time to make the transition back ... Return your attention to your surroundings ... feeling whatever you are sitting on ... listening to the sounds in this space ... and becoming more and more aware of your breath and your body ... When you are ready, stretch and open your eyes.

Heart Chakra / Anahata

Knowledge of the pure mind is obtained
by concentrating and meditating on the heart.

Yoga Sutra 3.35

Guided Imagery, Affirmations, and Healing Sound

Time: 15 minutes

Anahata is pronounced AH-nah-hot-ta

Summary: The fourth chakra is called the heart chakra. It is related to the lungs, heart, and arms. Although the physical heart is on the left side of the torso, the energy heart is in the center of the chest. It is associated with being able to love and be loved, as well as with being compassionate toward oneself and others. Forgiveness is the key to healing and balancing the fourth chakra and results in being nonjudgmental, feeling content, trusting, loving, and having a peaceful heart. Its color is predominantly green, and its sounds are Yam (pronounced Yum) and A (as in play).

Prepare yourself by sitting in an upright meditative position. Please make sure that your spine is straight. Close your eyes or keep them barely open.

Bring your attention to your breath and follow its pattern as you breathe in ... and out ... Allow your breath to become smooth ... and full ... breathing so that the inhalation and the exhalation are balanced.

Gradually, allow your exhalation to become longer than your inhalation ... Allowing this to happen is relaxing and centering.

Send your awareness to your arms, lungs, and heart. This is where the heart chakra is located. Take a few moments to explore and experience the sensations felt in your heart center.

Pause.

Maintain your awareness at the heart chakra and bring your attention back to your breath ... so now you are keeping your focus on your heart as well as on your breathing ... If your mind wanders, simply bring your attention back to your breath and to the heart charka ... If it's easier to maintain your awareness either on your breath or the heart chakra, choose one ... and allow your attention to settle there.

Pause.

Call to mind the color green ... sensing the color in any way you wish. Perhaps, imagine the color of the grass and trees in the spring ... perhaps an emerald ... In your mind's eye, allow the green image to become a green liquid or light ... or a green mist ... and imagine it within and around your heart ... sensing a cleansing green liquid ... a glowing light, or a healing mist in and around your heart.

Pause.

The heart chakra is associated with your right and responsibility to love and be loved ... Resolving and letting go of grief and forgiving oneself and others for loss, betrayal, and suffering is healthy and healing ... It is one of the heart chakra's lessons.

To help you integrate these lessons into your being, repeat the following statements aloud or silently.

"I have the right to love and be loved."

Pause. Repeat the affirmations every so often during the pause.

Notice what happens as you say these statements to yourself.

How do you react to this basic right?

Pause.

"I release and let go of grief."

"I forgive myself and others."

Pause.

"I am lovable."

"I am compassionate."

Pause.

This next part involves the use of sound. The sound of the fourth chakra is Yam *(pronounced as Yum with the Yu held longer than the m).* The Yam sound will send a healing sound to strengthen and balance your fourth chakra. First it will be said aloud; next it will be whispered; and finally it will be said silently. Each step will be repeated three times.

Now take a full breath in and repeat the sound of "Yam" out loud while exhaling ... Repeat the sound Yam over and over as you exhale, doing so for three breaths.

Breathe in … say Yam, Yam, Yam, Yam … while breathing out.

Repeat two more times.

Pause.

Continue whispering Yam for three breaths.

Pause long enough for this to take place.

Continue saying Yam silently for three breaths.

Pause long enough for this to take place.

Now let the Yam sound echo on by itself.

Pause.

The sound aaaaaaa *(as in play)* will continue to balance the fourth chakra and it will release and send the energy out to share.

This time, take a full breath and say a long aaaaaaa out loud for three breaths.

Pause long enough for this to take place.

Continue whispering aaaaaaa for three breaths.

Pause long enough for this to take place.

Continue saying aaaaaaa silently for three breaths.

Pause long enough for this to take place.

Now, let the aaaaaaa sound echo on by itself.

Pause.

Now, take some time on your own to focus on the location, color, lessons or sounds of the heart chakra … simply follow your own inclination … You could focus on the sensations at your heart center … the color green … or your right and responsibility to love and be loved … to release grief … to forgive … and be compassionate … Perhaps you would feel most at ease repeating Yam or aaaaaaa. Simply follow your own inclination for the next few minutes.

Longer pause.

It's time to make the transition back … Return your attention to your surroundings … feeling whatever you are sitting on … listening to the sounds in this space … and becoming more and more aware of your breath and your body … When you are ready, stretch and open your eyes.

Throat Chakra / Vissudha

*Cessation of hunger and thirst is obtained through concentration and medi-
tation on the hollow of the throat.*

Yoga Sutra 3.30

*Stillness in the meditation posture is achieved by concentration
and meditation on the throat.*

Yoga Sutra 3.31

Guided Imagery, Affirmations, and Healing Sound

Time: 15 minutes

Vissudha is pronounced vizh-SHOE-dah

Summary: The fifth chakra is the throat chakra. It is located in the area
of the throat, mouth, ears, as well as the hands. It is associated with
being willing to choose a self-expressive and creative life. Having a full,
resonant voice, being able to communicate clearly, being able to listen
to others, being truthful and choosing to align with the divine will are
signs of a balanced throat chakra. Its color is predominantly blue, and its
sounds are Ham (pronounced Hum) and E (like in speak).

Prepare yourself by sitting in an upright meditative position. Please make
sure that your spine is straight. Close your eyes or keep them barely open.

Bring your attention to your breath and follow its pattern as you
breathe in…and out…Allow your breath to become smooth…and
full…breathing so that the inhalation and the exhalation are balanced.

Gradually, allow your exhalation to become longer than your inhalation…Allowing this to happen is relaxing and centering.

Send your awareness to your throat, mouth and ears. This is where the
throat chakra is located. Take a few moments to explore and experience
the sensations felt in your throat chakra.

Pause.

Maintain your awareness at the throat chakra and bring your attention back to your breath ... so now you are keeping your focus on your throat as well as on your breathing ... If your mind wanders, simply bring your attention back to your breath and to the throat charka ... If it's easier to maintain your awareness either on your breath or the throat chakra, choose one ... and allow your attention to settle there.

Pause.

Call to mind the color blue ... sensing the color in any way you wish ... You might imagine the color of a clear blue sky ... or of a robin's egg ... perhaps a crystal blue sea ... In your mind's eye, allow the blue image to become a blue liquid, or light ... or mist ... and imagine it within and around your throat ... sensing a cleansing blue liquid ... a glowing light ... or a blue healing mist in and around your throat chakra.

Pause.

The throat chakra is associated with your right and responsibility to express yourself and to be heard based on your inner authority ... It is related to recognizing your true essence ... Letting go of dishonesty and being accountable for your actions is healthy and healing ... The throat chakra teaches that while you have the right and responsibility to be creative, you are accountable for the choices you make ... These are some of the throat chakra's lessons.

To help you integrate these lessons into your being, repeat the following statements aloud or silently.

"I express my self clearly."

"I have the right to be heard."

Pause. Repeat the affirmations every so often during the pause.

Notice what happens as you say these statements to yourself.

How do you react to these basic rights?

Pause.

"I release and let go of dishonesty."

Pause.

"I am creative."

Pause.

This next part involves the use of sound. The sound of the fifth chakra is Ham *(pronounced as Hum with the Hu held longer than the m)*. The sound of Ham will send a healing sound vibration to strengthen and balance your fifth chakra. First it will be said out loud; next it will be whispered; and finally it will be said silently. Each step will be repeated three times.

Now take a full breath in and repeat the sound of Ham out loud while exhaling... Repeat the sound Ham over and over as you exhale, doing so for three breaths.

Breathe in... say Ham, Ham, Ham, Ham... while breathing out.

Repeat two more times.

Pause.

Continue whispering Ham for three breaths.

Pause long enough for this to take place.

Continue saying Ham silently for three breaths.

Pause long enough for this to take place.

Now let the Ham sound echo on by itself.

Pause.

The sound eeeeeee (as in speak) will continue to balance the fifth chakra and it will release and send the energy out to share.

This time, take a full breath and say a long eeeeeee out loud for three breaths.

Pause long enough for this to take place.

Continue whispering eeeeeee for three breaths.

Pause long enough for this to take place.

Continue saying eeeeeee silently for three breaths.

Pause long enough for this to take place.

Now, let the eeeeeee sound echo on by itself.

Pause.

Now, take some time on your own to focus on the location, color, lessons or sounds of the throat chakra... Simply follow your own inclination... You could focus on the sensations at your throat... the color blue... your right and responsibility to express yourself and be heard... to listen... to release dishonesty... and be creative... Perhaps you would feel most at ease repeating Ham or eeeeeee. Simply follow your own inclination for the next few minutes.

Longer pause.

It's time to make the transition back ... Return your attention to your sur-roundings ... feeling whatever you are sitting on ... listening to the sounds in this space ... and becoming more and more aware of your breath and your body ... When you are ready, stretch and open your eyes.

Third Eye Chakra / Ajna

Everything can be clearly known with intuitive perception.
Yoga Sutra 3.33

Guided Imagery, Affirmations, and Healing Sound

Time: 15 minutes

Ajna is pronounced AAHJ-nah

Summary: The sixth chakra is the third eye chakra. It is located in the center of the forehead. It is associated with being insightful and intuitive. Being self-reflective and imaginative, as well as having a good memory, good dream recall, having a guiding vision for life, being able to recognize wisdom in any situation, and being observant to subtle signs that can guide are indicators of a balanced sixth chakra. Its color is predominantly indigo, and its sounds are Om and M.

Prepare yourself by sitting in an upright meditative position. Please make sure that your spine is straight. Close your eyes or keep them barely open.

Bring your attention to your breath and follow its pattern as you breathe in...and out...Allow your breath to become smooth...and full...breathing so that the inhalation and the exhalation are balanced.

Gradually, allow your exhalation to become longer than your inhalation...Allowing this to happen is relaxing and centering.

Send your awareness to the center of your forehead between your eyebrows. This is where the third eye chakra is located. Take a few moments to explore and experience the sensations felt in your third eye chakra.

Pause.

Maintain your awareness at the third eye chakra and bring your attention back to your breath...so now you are keeping your focus on your third eye as well as on your breathing...If your mind wanders, simply bring your attention back to your breath and to the third eye chakra...If it's easier to maintain your awareness either on your breath or the third eye chakra, choose one...and allow your attention to settle there.

Pause.

Call to mind the color indigo … sensing the color in any way you wish. It's a deep blue-violet … In your mind's eye, allow the indigo image to transform into an indigo liquid … light … or a misty indigo … and imagine it within and around your third eye … sensing a cleansing indigo liquid … a luminous light … or a healing mist in and around your third eye.

Pause.

The third eye chakra teaches that it is through opening the mind to wisdom, letting go of personalized beliefs, and purifying perceptions that your real spiritual intelligence is developed. It is important to be self-reflective and to learn how to watch, witness, and see the big picture … to let go of false truths and illusions … and to know that you have the right, responsibility and ability to access intuitive wisdom and universal truth.

To help you integrate these lessons into your being, repeat the following statements aloud or silently.

"I have the right and responsibility to see the big picture."

"I have the right to be intuitive."

Pause. Repeat the affirmations every so often during the pause.

Notice what happens as you say these statements to yourself.

How do you react to these basic rights?

Pause.

"I release and let go of illusion."

Pause.

"My intuition is trustworthy and I follow my inner wisdom."

Pause.

This next part involves the use of sound. The sound of the sixth chakra is Om *(pronounced as Om with the ooo held longer than the m)*. The sound of Om will send a healing sound vibration to strengthen and balance your sixth chakra. First it will be said out loud; next it will be whispered; and finally it will be said silently. Each step will be repeated three times.

Now take a full breath in, and repeat the sound of Om out loud while exhaling … Repeat the sound Om over and over as you exhale, doing so for three breaths.

Breathe in … say Om, Om, Om, Om … while breathing out.

Repeat two more times.

Pause.

Continue whispering Om for three breaths.

Pause long enough for this to take place.

Continue saying Om silently for three breaths.

Pause long enough for this to take place.

Now let the Om sound echo on by itself.

Pause.

The sound mmmmmmm will continue to balance the sixth chakra and it will release and send the energy out to share.

This time, take a full breath and say a long mmmmmmm out loud for three breaths.

Pause long enough for this to take place.

Continue whispering mmmmmmm for three breaths.

Pause long enough for this to take place.

Continue saying mmmmmmm silently for three breaths.

Pause long enough for this to take place.

Now, let the mmmmmmm sound echo on by itself.

Pause.

Now, take some time on your own to focus on the location, color, lessons or sounds of the third eye chakra... Simply follow your own inclination... You could focus on the sensations at your third eye... the color indigo... your right and responsibility to be insightful... to release illusion... to be watchful... and to witness... Perhaps; you would feel most at ease repeating Om or mmmmmmm. Simply follow your own inclination for the next few minutes.

Longer pause.

It's time to make the transition back... Return your attention to your surroundings... feeling whatever you are sitting on... listening to the sounds in this space... and becoming more and more aware of your breath and your body... When you are ready, stretch and open your eyes.

Crown Chakra / Sahasrara

Visions and revelations of the masters and enlightened beings are obtained through concentration and meditation on the crown of the head.

Yoga Sutra 3.33

Guided Imagery, Affirmations, and Healing Sound

Time: 15 minutes

Sahasrara is pronounced SAH-has-rar-ah

Summary: The seventh chakra is the crown chakra. It is located at the top and slightly above the head in the area of the fontanel, the soft spot found on babies' heads. It is associated with awakening cosmic consciousness, wisdom, and spirituality through prayer, meditation, and devotion. A balanced crown chakra is associated with having a crystal clear mind, cultivating awareness without thoughts, and being connected to unlimited individual spiritual experience. Likewise, it is being able to question, assimilate, and analyze information, and to be totally present in the here and now. Its color can be either predominantly violet or white and its sound is NG (as in wing). Ultimately it is beyond sound.

Prepare yourself by sitting in an upright meditative position. Please make sure that your spine is straight. Close your eyes or keep them barely open.

Bring your attention to your breath and follow its pattern as you breathe in... and out... Allow your breath to become smooth... and full... breathing so that the inhalation and the exhalation are balanced.

Gradually, allow your exhalation to become longer than your inhalation... Allowing this to happen is relaxing and centering.

Send your awareness to the top of your head. This is where the crown chakra is located. Take a few moments to explore and experience the sensations felt in your crown chakra.

Pause.

Maintain your awareness at the crown chakra and bring your attention back to your breath... so now you are keeping your focus on the top of your head as well as on your breathing... If your mind wanders, simply bring your attention back to your breath and to the crown charka... If it's easier to maintain your awareness either on your breath or the crown chakra, choose one... and allow your attention to settle there.

Pause.

Call to mind the color violet... sensing the color in any way you wish. You might imagine the color of a freshly opened violet... the ultra-violet light that naturally occurs at twilight... anything that is a pale purple... In your mind's eye, allow the violet image to transform into a violet liquid... light... or mist... and imagine it within and around the top of your head... sensing a cleansing violet liquid... a luminous light... or a healing mist in and around your crown chakra.

Pause.

The crown chakra teaches that our true nature is as a divine being... Limitless devotion to that awakening of oneself and others is profoundly wise and the spiritually connected path home... Resolving and letting go of attachments to who and what you are and aren't is healthy and healing... and reveals your true, divine nature.

To help you integrate these lessons into your being, repeat the following statements aloud or silently.

"I have the right be intelligent."

Pause. Repeat the affirmations every so often during the pause.

Notice what happens as you say this statement to yourself.

How do you react to these basic rights?

Pause.

"I release and let go of attachments."

Pause.

"I am wise."

"I am connected spiritually."

Pause.

"I am divine."

This next part involves the use of sound. The sound of the seventh chakra is "nnnnggggg" *(as in wing)*. The sound of "nnnnggg" will send a healing sound vibration to balance your seventh chakra. First it will be said out loud; next it will be whispered; and finally it will be said silently. Each step will be repeated three times.

Now take a full breath in and repeat the sound of nnnngggg out loud while exhaling.

Pause long enough for this to take place.

Continue whispering nnnngggg for three breaths.

Pause long enough for this to take place.

Continue saying nnnngggg silently for three breaths.

Pause long enough for this to take place.

Now, let the nnnngggg sound echo on by itself.

Pause.

The crown chakra is beyond sound. Allow your mind to become crystal clear... letting go of your thoughts and being aware of an inner silence... pure awareness without thinking thoughts. When thoughts come in, label them "thinking" and return your attention to the quiet.

Pause.

Now, take some time on your own to focus on the location, color, lessons, or sounds of the crown chakra... Simply follow your own inclination... You could focus on the sensations at your crown... the color vioet... your divine connection... to release attachments... Perhaps; you would feel most at ease repeating nnnnggg or dwelling in silence. Simply follow your own inclination for the next few minutes.

Longer pause.

It's time to make the transition back... Return your attention to your surroundings... feeling whatever you are sitting on... listening to the sounds in this space... and becoming more and more aware of your breath and your body... When you are ready, stretch and open your eyes.

Hatha Yoga Postures
to Awaken the Chakras

The practice of hatha yoga is well known for improving flexibility and strength and for having a positive impact on the body-mind. As important and powerful as this is, the essential benefits extend far deeper into our essence as human beings through the influence the postures have on the chakras: physically, psycho-energetically and spiritually.

From the earliest beginnings of the tradition, certain postures have been recognized as being particularly powerful and effective for opening, aligning and balancing the chakras individually and as a whole. Many of these postures are listed on the chakra chart. Please consult a qualified yoga teacher or refer to instructional materials on hatha yoga for further information and instructions for the postures.

To help get you started, several postures are described and illustrated on the pages that follow. More are listed on the Chakra Chart. The postures have been selected for their unique effect on each chakra and sequenced to maximize their integrated benefit. To optimize your experience, it is recommended that these postures be practiced in the order as presented. However, if you choose a different sequence, simply notice the effect it has on your experience.

Here are a few recommendations for your yoga practice.

- Choose a well-ventilated room with no distractions. Turn the phone and pager off.

- Wear comfortable clothing and use a yoga mat, blanket, or large towel for cleanliness, comfort, and safety.

- Allow 2–3 hours after a big meal and 1 hour after a snack. Otherwise, you may be uncomfortable, and you will not feel the subtle effects of the practice.

- Always stretch and limber up before doing yoga poses. Consult a yoga teacher or instructional materials for ideas. Move slowly and avoid hasty or jerky movements.

- Never force a position. Listen to your body and let your body form the pose at its own pace. This is one of the secrets of yoga.

- Breathe fully and consciously at all times to balance and nourish your body, mind, and heart. Breathing deeply develops focus enabling you to experience the essence and presence of yoga.

- Hold each pose for as long as you can breathe easily and deeply and remain steady and comfortable. Respond to the signals from your body, and always avoid painful stretches, especially in your joints.

- Props to help with your comfort in the poses include:

  Yoga mat, blanket, or beach towel

  Two firm cushions

  Pillows of various sizes

  Yoga strap or neck tie

  Bath towel (roll it up and hold it with two rubber bands)

- To benefit fully, it is best to do yoga on a regular basis. Ten minutes every day is much better than practicing sporadically.

- Join a yoga class taught by a qualified, certified teacher for the best experience.

- People with health conditions should consult their health care professional before practicing this hatha yoga routine.

1. Root Chakra

Child / Garbasana or Balasana.

Pronounced gar-BAH-sah-nah or bahl-AH-sah-nah

1. Kneel on the floor with your shins and the tops of your feet on the floor. Lower your hips to your heels. For greater comfort, place a pillow over your calves and a small rolled towel under your ankles as needed.

2. Bend forward from your hips and lower your chest to your knees. Widen the distance between your knees to make room for the front of your body and to keep your hips near your heels.

3. Rest your forehead on the floor. If necessary, place a small pillow under your forehead for support.

4. Extend your arms on the floor in front of you with your palms down. Another position for your arms is at your sides, your hands near your feet with your palms up.

5. Focus your attention at the base of your spine, where your body meets the ground (shins, forehead, arms, and hands), and your adrenal glands.

6. Rest while breathing deeply and hold as long as comfortable.

7. When ready, lift back up.

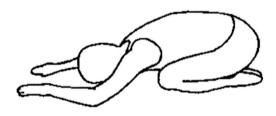

2. Sacral Chakra

Cat Pose / Bidalasana

Pronounced bee-doll-AH-sah-nah

1. Start on your hands and knees.
2. Place your hands under and no wider than your shoulders. If necessary, move your hands forward to take pressure off your wrists. Place your knees directly under your hips.
3. Align your back so the natural curves at the low back and behind the neck are present.
4. Focus your attention on your pelvis, low back, abdomen, and reproductive glands throughout the following movements.
5. Exhale through your nose; tuck your tailbone under; round your back like a Halloween cat; and lower your chin to your throat.
6. Inhale through your nose and lift your tailbone; then lift your chest and finally your head.
7. Repeat steps five and six for five to ten breaths.

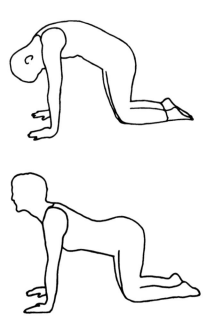

3. Solar Plexus Chakra

Boat / Navasana

Pronounced nah-VAH-sah-nah

1. Lie down on your belly and place your knees and feet almost together.
2. Place your arms and hands on the floor beside you. Palms down.
3. Press your pelvic triangle (two hip bones and pubic bone) toward the floor and raise your upper body, legs, and feet. Your arms rest near or on the floor.
4. Focus your attention on your solar plexus, pancreas, and adrenal glands.
5. Breathe long, slow, deep breaths through your nose. Hold as long as comfortable.
6. When ready, exhale while slowly lowering back to the ground.

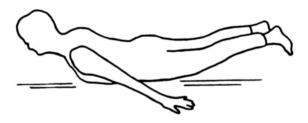

4. Heart Chakra

Bridge / Setu Bandhasana

Pronounced SAY-too bhan-DAH-sah-nah

1. Lie on your back on the floor.
2. Bend your knees and place your feet on the floor below your knees. Keep your knees and feet hip-width apart throughout the pose.
3. Stretch your arms out beside your torso on the floor.
4. Exhale and press your feet down into the floor as you lift your hips up. Lift your spine off the floor one vertebra at a time.
5. When your hips are raised as high as is comfortable press your sternum away from your pubic bone. Clasp your hands under your body and gain more shoulder support by scooting your shoulder blades closer together.
6. Focus your attention on your heart, lungs, and thymus gland.
7. Breathe long, slow, deep breaths through your nose. Remain in the position for as long as comfortable.
8. Slowly move your arms apart. Exhale and gently lower your back to the floor, one vertebra at a time.

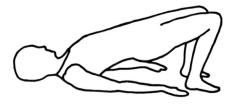

5. Throat Chakra

Supported Fish / Matsyasana

Pronounced mahtz-YAH-sah-nah

1. Lie down on your back. If necessary, place a pillow under your knees for support.
2. Place another firm pillow lengthwise under your shoulders. Allow your head to tip backward slightly, and your chin to lift up, stretching your throat. Place a small rolled towel so it lightly supports the back of your head if needed.
3. Rest your arms by your sides.
4. Breathe deeply while focusing on your throat, neck, and thyroid gland. Remain in the position as long as you are comfortable.
5. To release, gently roll to your side and rest.
6. Press your hands into the floor and sit up.

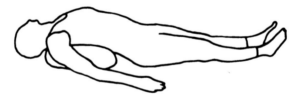

6. Third Eye Chakra

Spinal Twist / Matysendrasana

Pronounced mahtz-yen-DRAH-sah-nah

1. Sit cross-legged on the floor with your spine erect. If necessary, sit on a firm cushion to raise your hips so they are higher than your knees. Otherwise, sit on a chair.
2. Place your left hand on the outside of your right knee.
3. Circle your right shoulder up, back and down and place your right hand on the floor (or chair seat) next to your right hip.
4. Exhale and gently and very slowly turn your low back, ribs, shoulder, neck, head, and eyes to the right. Do not use force.
5. Lengthen your spine each time you inhale, and gently deepen your rotation each time you exhale.
6. Focus your attention on your forehead and your pineal and pituitary glands. Breathe slowly, deeply, and evenly.
7. To release, lift your right hand off the floor or chair seat and very slowly turn your torso back around to face the front.
8. Repeat the twist on the other side.

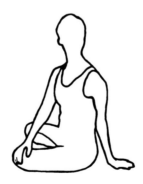

7. Crown Chakra

Yoga Seal / Yoga Mudra

Pronounced Yoga MOO-drah

1. Sit cross-legged on the floor with your spine erect. If necessary, sit on a firm cushion to raise your hips up so they are higher than your knees. You may also place small pillows under your knees for support. Otherwise, sit on a chair.

2. Clasp your right wrist with your left hand behind your back. If needed, hold a strap or tie between your hands.

3. Close your eyes.

4. Exhale through your nose. Lengthen your spine and slowly bend forward from your hips. Lead with your sternum instead of your head. Lower forward as far as comfortable and relax.

7. Focus your attention on the crown of your head and breathe slowly, deeply and evenly. Remain in the position as long as you are comfortable.

8. Release very slowly. Breathe in and slowly lift up about one third of the way. Exhale and let yourself naturally sink down a bit. Inhale while rising up another third of the way. Exhale. Inhale while rising up the rest of the way. The secret is in coming up as slowly as possible.

9. Release your hands and rest them on your lap.

10. Sit quietly and notice the uplifting, peaceful feeling.

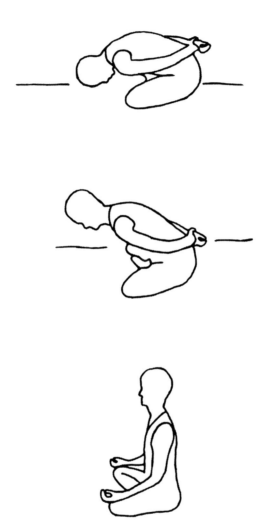

Yoga Meditation Practices
Paradise Present

Concentrating your whole mind on a single object
will soon purify your mind.

Bhagavad Gita 6.12

What is subtle and hidden from view can be realized through
concentration, meditation, and absolute contemplation.

Yoga Sutra 3.25

When someone is absorbed in dreamless sleep,
he is one with the Self, though he knows it not.

Chandogya Upanishad VI.8.1

Meditation is practiced for all sorts of purposes ranging from its ability to lower blood pressure to reaching enlightenment. Meditation is the general term used to refer to both the practice of meditation techniques and to the various states achieved through meditation, both mental and nonmental. Similarly, the expression "going to sleep" is the general term that refers to all the stages of sleep from getting ready for bed to deep sleep.

You are already familiar with the sleep process of getting tired, preparing for sleep, falling asleep, perhaps dreaming, being in the dreamless zone, and eventually waking up. Similarly, there are stages of meditation as well as a process to follow. This process includes setting the intention to meditate, taking a sitting position that facilitates meditation, practicing a technique to settle the restless mind, noticing distracting thoughts, returning your attention to your technique, and gradually developing the ability to focus your attention for longer periods of time. Eventually, a state is experienced in which the meditation technique is no longer needed, and the mind becomes quiet and peaceful as the heart naturally opens. This deeper stage of meditation is a nonthinking, nonemotional state, yet one in which you are attentive and awake. It often feels spacious, and the boundaries of time disappear. Simply put, the Yoga Sutras define these stages as asana (taking a comfortable seat), pranayama breathing (a technique used to settle the mind), pratyahara (sense withdrawal), dharana (concentration), dhyana (meditation), and samadhi (transcendence).

Before getting into this deeper state of meditation, our minds try to pull us away through distracting thoughts, feelings, and sensations. As in the stages of sleep, we go back and forth between the dreaming and nondreaming stages. In meditation, it is normal to go back and forth between having a wandering mind and clearing and focusing the mind with the meditation technique, the conscious return to the technique, and experiencing a settled mind without having to rely on the meditation technique.

Meditation is different from guided imagery. While guided imagery uses the mind to direct and focus itself on various subject areas and encourages mental images, thoughts, and feelings to occur, meditation cultivates nonmental awareness. Meditation, however, often uses guided imagery (a mental process) as a starting point in this process. Experientially, meditation teaches us to develop a state of awareness that is not limited to thoughts but rather is impartial to and not identified with whatever thoughts arise. This gradually evolves into equanimity, the ability to remain compassionate, sensitive, highly aware, yet uninvolved in the activities of the mind, emotions, and senses. Equanimity enables us to open ourselves to new vistas of experience, living our lives to the fullest. Ultimately, the goal of meditation is to know and remember the experience of yoga, or union, between oneself and the divine.

Here are a few yoga practices and meditation methods to focus the mind and reawaken the divine connection.

Namaste'

Journey to the Core (12-15 minutes)

Gazing / Trā taka (10 to 30 minutes)

My Thoughts are Made of Consciousness (10 to 20 minutes)

The Inner Eye of Awareness (15 to 20 minutes)

Om Mantra or Chant (variable time)

Om Meditation (15 or more minutes)

Japa - Om Mantra Repetition (variable time)

Mindfulness (15 to 25 minutes)

Walking Meditation (15 to 60 minutes)

Namaste'

Yoga Practice

Namaste' is pronounced nah-mah-STAY.

Namaste' is a sign of respect and means "I honor the divine light that shines in me, and I honor the divine light that shines in you," or "the spirit in me honors the spirit in you." Namaste' was referred to in the Mahabharata, an epic poem from ancient India that comes to us from between 2000 and 3000 years ago. To this day, it is used as a gesture to greet others as well as to say good-bye.

The practice is to bring the palms and fingers together in front of your heart in the prayer position while giving a nod of your head to the person being acknowledged. This hand gesture is also called Namaskar or Anjali Mudra.

Namaste' is often used at the beginning or end of a yoga or meditation session to unite the group, generate respect, and remember the divine connection.

Deepak Chopra recommends saying Namaste' to yourself silently when first making eye contact with people. In this case, the hand gesture is omitted. Try it and notice what happens.

Journey to the Core

Guided Imagery Practice

Contributed by Christopher Baxter

Time: 12 to 15 minutes

Summary: This practice accomplishes several interconnected goals. First, it helps to structurally open and expand the respiratory activity of the torso, belly, and back, giving us an open door into the core. Next, the use of sound facilitates the release of habitual emotional tension in those areas as the sounding gives the nervous system a message that "all is well, it's safe to let go, I can relax now." This helps us move into a felt, sensory awareness of our core.

Deeper in, it sets up a safe space, filled with sensation, that encourages the natural curiosity of our mind to drop from superficial thinking into deeply feeling the interior spaciousness of the body. We feel our biological life through the contrast between intense sensations (when the breath is intentionally held) and the release into deep stillness (when the breath spontaneously pauses). As we learn how to enter and roam through the interior of our body, we notice how "at home," stable, comfortable, and intuitive we are. An inner knowing, or mindfulness, arises. This intimate, touching awareness is grounded in the core of the physical frame of our body. It is not an abstract, disembodied, remote higher consciousness. Finally, when we rest in this core of awareness, rooted in our body, we have no doubt as to who we are. We directly perceive our Self as the reality of this moment.

Background Notes: In yoga, our deepest self is reached through an integration of practices that network body, mind, heart, and emotions into a coherent awareness — an awareness rooted in our core. This expanded awareness is paradoxically developed through a concentrated application of yogic techniques. Gradually, what begins as a focused, technical practice evolves into a spontaneous, expanding process. In other words, we shift from using a time-tested method, to being guided by an evolutionary, unprecedented awakening — all set in motion by the yogic practices.

As a deeper awareness of our true nature intuitively unfolds from the inside out, our way of being attentive moves beyond mental thinking and into nonmental awareness — or mindfulness. During practice, as we shift our emphasis to the inner world, withdrawing from the outer world, we gradually leave behind the familiar reference points of our culture, our thoughts and even our identity as a personality. This can be very disorienting to the conditioned mind. Therefore, to support us in making this subtle, inward journey, it is vital that we feel safe and stable.

A stable anchor for this exploration into the unknown is the ability to trust our inner self. The key here is to find, feel, and relax into our core. What is meant by core? Think of it as a multidimensional presence.

Physically, we can speak of the core as the central axis of the torso, the gravitational plumb line that drops from the center of the skull to the center of the pelvic floor.

Structurally, the spine and pelvic bowel is the core of the skeletal body, whereas our deep pelvic, abdominal, diaphragmatic, and thoracic muscles are our muscular core.

Neurologically, the dural tube is the core — a hollow cable running through the spine that carries the central nervous system.

The core of breathing is considered to be the gap, or Madhya, between the in and out breath — when respiration ceases and metabolic activity is at a minimum.

Likewise, the core of the mind is known to be the gap between thoughts, when all that prevails is profound stillness.

Energetically, according to the yogic tradition, core can be considered as the kanda, or storehouse of our life force, situated in the subtle body approximately three fingers below the navel. The kanda can be visualized as a root ball of swirling energy in which the sushumna nadi, like an energy stalk, is rooted. From here it extends up through the subtle body. It is from this energy stalk that each of the seven chakras, like flowers of energy on tiny stems, branch off.

Spiritually we may call our core the soul, or even our heart – our center of love, personal awareness and infinite divinity.

From a quantum physics perspective, we can consider our core as an expanding spaciousness, devoid of any matter whatsoever, intelligent energy moving in endless, unfathomable patterns.

When we speak of core, it refers to these and other subtler dimensions.

Materials: small cushion, eye bag or small towel over the eyes, small rolled hand towel, journal and pen.

Practice of Journeying into Your Core

Come into a position lying comfortably on your back. Perhaps place a cushion behind your knees and a small rolled hand towel under the curve of your neck.

Bring your hands to rest on your belly and begin to notice the movement of breath in your belly. Focus on your exhalation. As you exhale pull in your belly slowly, yet firmly towards your spine. As you inhale, expand your belly up. Repeat this a few times, feeling the sensation in your belly and breath.

Now begin to add a soft sighing sound to your exhalations, the kind of sigh you might make as you settle into an easy chair at the end of a hard day.

Notice any changes — emotionally ... energetically ... physically. Repeat this sigh a dozen times or so, as long as it feels comfortable.

Pause.

Do you notice a lessening of tension and an increase in awareness? ... Do you notice that your sense of self is dropping out of your skull and centering in your chest or belly? ... Do you feel perhaps a safety or unusual confidence in the moment?

Shift your hands to your ribs and exhale. Then with a willful contraction of your chest muscles, feel your ribs tighten even more against your torso. Breathe in and expand.

Again after a few rounds, add the sounding sigh. Repeat a dozen times or so.

Pause.

What is happening now? ... What do you feel? ... Where in your body do you now feel your center of awareness is located? ... Can you feel your center of attention shifting into your ribs? ... Do you notice if you are dropping away from the surface?

Now with hands on your breastbone, repeat this breathing technique about a dozen times.

Pause.

Do you notice your chest more vividly? ... Not just the surface but the heart and the inner chest as well ... the sensations ... the presence ... the intelligence ... Are you aware of emotions moving ... or energy streaming?

Now sandwich your hands between your back and the floor. Again, repeat the physical technique and pause.

Again notice the effect on your awareness, identity, or sense of self.

Release your hands from behind your back and rest them at your sides.

Finally, slowly begin an overall exhalation...simultaneously pull your belly, ribs, sternum, and back snugly into the central core of your body. Briefly and easily hold your breath out; do not strain. Then slowly inhale and expand your belly, ribs, chest, and back. Briefly and easily hold the breath in, do not strain. Then, with a long, slow sounding sigh...release.

Repeat this process three or so times.

Pause.

Release all the techniques, let go of controlling your breath, and notice what now happens spontaneously...how your breath rises, and falls, and stops...all on its own. Notice how you perceive who you are...how thinking is less dominant and feeling awareness more prominent.

Relax into the steadiness and comfort this brings, particularly when your breath stops on its own...Let that easy, steady, breathless state expand and enjoy the core stillness it brings. Do you feel more restful, more joyful?

Reflect deeply on this and recognize the awareness of an inner presence and aliveness that is here, waiting for you as you let go of control.

Notice how comforted you feel...and how secure...and how stable you really are...deep inside.

Can you sense a confidence and trust in the ease of the moment...and can you allow that to radiate from the anchoring point in your core, all the way back to the surface of your mind, body, and emotions? Enjoy this journey to the core for a few more moments and then, as you are ready, bring your awareness back to the room.

Once reoriented, take a few moments and journal any awarenesses that have occurred for you, paying close attention to the sense of writing from the internal spaciousness within.

Author's note: Christopher Baxter, president of AtmaYoga Educational Services, has been a practitioner of yoga since 1971. He was a founding member of Kripalu Center, which for 20 years has been one of the most widely known and respected yoga training facilities in the world.

Christopher is the author of *Kripalu Hatha Yoga* and was instrumental in the development of Kripalu Yoga and the Kripalu Yoga Teacher Training methodology.

Christopher is committed to spreading the teachings of yoga through a unique method he developed named AtmaYoga: A Compassionate Way to the Core Self. Two Eastern traditions he has spent many years practicing and studying, yoga and Buddhism, are integrated with a comprehensive western approach to anatomy and physiology. The result is a practice that is anatomically sound, physically and energetically alive, and deeply contemplative.

For more information on his classes, workshops and yoga teacher training program, visit www.atmayoga.com or call 904 687 8482

Gazing / Trātaka

Meditation

Trātaka is pronounced TRAH-tahk

Time: 10 to 20 minutes

Summary: Trātaka is effective for focusing an overly active mind. The wandering mind is quickly settled by gazing steadily at an object. The eyes alternate between focusing outwardly with the eyes open and inwardly with the eyes closed. Anything can be looked at that absorbs your attention and fosters peaceful and inspiring feelings. The flame of a candle, a flower, stone, or an inspiring symbol or photo is commonly used. A scented candle engages the sense of smell. Ancient yogis claimed this meditation technique cures all eye afflictions and leads to clairvoyance. According to the *Hatha Yoga Pradipika*, the purpose of gazing is to arouse the internal vision and to make the vision steady by stopping the eye movements. Doing so unites and integrates the brain and the eyes.

> *"Looking intently with an unwavering gaze at a small point*
> *until tears are shed is known as Trātaka by the acharyas (teachers).*
> *Trātaka eradicates all eye diseases, fatigue and sloth*
> *and closes the doorway creating these problems.*
> *It should be carefully kept secret like a golden casket."*
> Hatha Yoga Pradipika, II.31-32 (written around 1200 a.d.)

Begin by placing an object for meditation at eye level and two to three feet away.

Sit in a manner suitable for meditation with your spine erect...your shoulders back and down...your hands resting on your lap...your sternum gently lifting...and your neck and head balanced...Restfully, close your eyes.

Release muscular tension in your body by scanning your awareness throughout your body, beginning at your feet and working your way up to the crown of your head. Acknowledge the muscles that are comfortable and those that are tense...Permit the muscles that are tight to soften and relax...perhaps by sending a soothing stream of air or light into the tightness to loosen it ... or perhaps by squeezing the muscle even more and then allowing it to soften and relax ... or by giving it mental permission to relax and let go.

Now, focus your attention on your breath. Follow the air as it goes in and as it leaves ... When your mind wanders, gently bring your attention to your breath ... breathing in and out ... smoothly and naturally.

Pause.

Slowly open your eyes about halfway and in a way that feels soft and easy. Gently begin softly gazing at the object you have chosen ... As your eyes wander away, shift them back to your object.

Hold your eyes open as long as possible. Hold them open until they water, have to blink, or become uncomfortable (2-5 minutes).

When you have to, close them softly and restfully ... Now, watch the image as it appears in your mind's eye ... softly gazing inwardly ... If the image moves, bring it back to the center ... When you notice your mind commenting on the image ... tenderly bring your attention back to the image itself.

When the image begins to fade, open your eyes and begin gazing at the external object once again.

Continue this sequence, gazing outwardly and inwardly, alternating between the external object and the internal image ... flowing back and forth.

See if you can let go of all your thoughts and feelings as you simply gaze back and forth ... Take your time; there's no need to rush ... remaining fully aware, without having to think.

Once the image stabilizes, study it, looking intently ... If your mind begins to comment on the object, release the thoughts and return to gazing.

Notice the feeling of tranquility, serenity, and inner stillness ... absorbed in the peace and quiet.

Pause.

With your eyes closed, bring the palms of your hands together and feel them touch ... begin to rub your hands together briskly ... feel the warmth and energy as you continue rubbing your hands together ... now, slowly cup your hands and carefully place them gently over your closed eyes ... Feel the sensations of your cupped hands as they cover your eyes ... soothing and comforting your eyes ... Feel free to gently massage your forehead and temples with your fingers.

When you feel ready to finish this experience, with your hands still cupped over your eyes, begin blinking your eyes open, allowing the light and the sight to filter in ... Gradually lower your hands to your lap and open your eyes up more and more.

Breathe, stretch, and mindfully notice how you feel deep inside.

Author's note: The Meditation on the Universal Light, by Nischala Joy Devi, combines candle gazing with expanding the heart.

My Thoughts are Made of Consciousness
Working with the Mind:
The Energy behind Thinking

Guided Meditation and Practice

Contributed by Sally Kempton

Time: 10 to 20 minutes

This practice can be a meditation in itself; yet it is most transformative when we use it along with our other meditation practices as a way of dealing with distracting or intrusive thoughts and mental static. Its power lies in the fact that it allows us to integrate our thoughts into our meditation, rather than looking at thoughts as obstructions or becoming distracted by them.

To be fully effective, this practice needs to become natural and automatic, so I recommend working with it over a period of time and making it a conscious part of your daily meditation routine. In time you'll notice that it is genuinely changing the way you hold thoughts. It is one of the most effective ways there is to stop identifying yourself with the thoughts that pass through the mind.

The teaching behind the practice comes from the Shaiva tantras, a group of sophisticated and comparatively modern yogic texts that appeared in northern India around the 9th century and remained relatively secret until about 50 years ago. The teaching is simple: everything that appears in your mind is made of consciousness or awareness or, if you like, mind-energy. Your thoughts and feelings are all made of the same subtle, invisible, highly dynamic "stuff." It's so evanescent that it can dissolve in a moment, yet it's so powerful that it can create imagined realities that run you for a lifetime. The amazing thing about this energy, the stuff of thoughts, is that if you recognize it for what it is, it will no longer trouble you. In short, if we look at thoughts and feelings with the recognition that they are all made of consciousness, of awareness, of energy, they stop being obstructive.

Most of us ignore what our thoughts are really made of. Instead, we focus on their content and implicitly believe that thought content is important and real. In fact, thought content is simply the shape or form that thought energy is taking. There's an energetic dance going on inside your mind, and instead of seeing the dance itself, we're getting caught up in the story.

So, in this practice, instead of getting caught up in the content, we let go of it, and investigate the energetic substance of a thought. We simply look into the energy that the thought is made of, the actual substance of the thought itself.

My Thoughts are Made of Consciousness

Sit quietly, focusing your attention on the movement of your breath as it flows in and out of your nostrils. Let your breath be your anchor.

As your mind entrains itself to your breath, begin to notice the thoughts passing through your mind. The mind is so perverse that sometimes, when you do this, your stream of consciousness might suddenly come to a halt, which is all to the good. But for now, in order to understand the practice, you might even create a thought. Let it be a sweet thought — a beach or the name of someone you like.

Hold the thought for a few seconds. Now, focus on the thought's substance. Look at what the thought is made of. Notice the energetic or feeling space the thought creates inside your mind.

If you like, you can formally label the thought. Name it "consciousness," "energy," or "thought-stuff" just as, if you were practicing mindfulness meditation, you might label it "thinking."

Notice what happens to the thoughts when you recognize what they are made of.

Return to your breath. Each time a thought arises, recognize it as energy. Notice the space in your mind that arises when you do this. Focus on that inner spaciousness for a moment. Let yourself relax into the space inside your own mind.

Author's note: Sally Kempton wrote *The Heart of Meditation: Pathways to a Deeper Experience* under her former monastic name of Swami Durgananda. Her book is one of my favorites on meditation, and I recommend it highly. One of today's most experienced and knowledgable meditation teachers, Sally has been practicing for thirty years, many of them as a disciple of meditation masters Swami Muktananda and Gurumayi Chidvilasananda. A former senior teacher of Siddha Yoga meditation, Sally teaches workshops in meditation and spiritual awareness in the US, Europe and South America, and writes a column, "Inner Life," for *Yoga Journal*. Her schedule appears on her website, www.sallykempton.com.

The Inner Eye of Awareness

Guided Meditation

Time: 15-20 minutes

Summary: This meditation opens the door to your inner awareness and to a place of deep inner stillness by focusing your awareness upon the inner pulsation that is seen behind the closed eyes. Yogis have used this practice for thousands of years.

Begin by settling yourself in a meditation posture that is comfortable for you. This may be sitting upright on a firm chair or on the floor with or without a meditation cushion. Choose a position that allows your spine to be upright and erect, respecting your knees, hips, shoulders, and back.

Refine your seat by settling more firmly onto your sitz bones... Level your pelvis... Circle your shoulders up, back and down... Lift your sternum... Place your chin so it's parallel to the floor... And lift the crown of your head gently upwards.

Place your hands either on your lap, one hand cradled in the other with your thumbs touching or place one on each knee and touch the pads of your thumbs to the tip of your index fingers. Your hands can face up or down.

Speaking from your heart, quietly set an intention by saying something like, "I'm going to be still for 15 minutes, focusing my consciousness. As soon as I notice I'm thinking or distracted, I will let go of the distraction and return to my consciousness."

Take a few moments to get in touch with the sensations present in your body... Ask for and receive permission from your body to meditate.

Get in touch with your thinking mind... and your emotions... Ask for and receive permission from your mind... and emotions to meditate.

Ask for help and grace from your inner teacher and your connection to the divine (Jesus, Buddha, the Divine Mother, etc.).

Follow your breath for a few minutes, or use whatever method works best for becoming centered.

Take a moment to offer your meditation to be of benefit to all sentient beings.

With your outer eyes closed, become aware of your inner eye by looking at what you see behind your eyelids... turning your attention inward to your consciousness... Simply observe your own inner world with your inner eye so you can become more aware of what you actually see behind your closed eyes... Perhaps you see a field of gray... or a mosaic of color... something like the night sky... a ruby red... or a bluish-gray light... The shapes and colors you see doesn't matter at all. What's important is to impartially watch whatever you see as you see it.

You are looking at mind stuff... the inner consciousness... this is the place from which all thoughts, feelings, perceptions, and sensations arise and subside. It's the energetic ground.

If you would like to spark your inner experience, blink your eyes tighter, even though they are already closed, and pay attention to what you see... Another way is to rub your eyes through your closed eyelids very softly and tenderly.

Now notice the dynamic quality of this inner consciousness... Notice if what you see constantly shifts and changes, forming new patterns of subtle movement... a kind of dance of images... color... or shapes... vibrating and pulsing... expanding and contracting... This is your inner consciousness... It's made of energy... Merely watch the pulsation and its ongoing nature.

Take as much time as you wish to follow the patterns of the coming and going of the designs that are a part of your inner world of awareness.

Pause.

When you notice that your mind has drifted into thinking, bring your awareness back to looking behind your eyelids.

Pause.

If you would like to deepen your experience, find a point of inner awareness that captures your attention right now and in this moment... Perhaps it's a darker or maybe a brighter spot... and focus there... watching and witnessing... and allowing it to take you inward still... and deeper.

Pause.

It's time to make the transition back... Bring your attention back to your breath and without changing it, follow along with your mind's eye ... following the inhalation and exhalation and the coming and going of your breath.

Pause.

Focus your attention on the rest of your body ... shift your weight ... and stretch a little bit ... and return to being still.

Pause.

Open your eyes just a sliver and then close them, returning inside for a little longer ... Slowly blink your eyes open, aware of blending your inner sight with the outer world ... Sit a bit longer and gradually open your eyes and stretch more fully. Notice any changes that have happened since your inward journey into the eye of consciousness.

Author's Note: This practice is one I discovered on my own as a little girl. Recently, I returned to this form of meditation and found it to be particularly effective for capturing my attention and holding me in the moment. This rendition was inspired by Sally Kempton and her book *The Heart of Meditation: Pathways to a Deeper Experience*, published by the SYDA Foundation in 2002. Sally shares a wealth of her vast knowledge and experience in her book, which is one of my favorites.

Om Mantra or Chant

Guided Meditation

Time: 8 to 10 minutes to learn. The practice length is variable

Summary: Om is a powerful sound vibration, considered as sacred, that has been meditated on silently or chanted aloud for well over 5000 years. It is said to be a universal mantra and serves as the root sound for Amen and Shalom. In fact, yogis claim it is the root sound for all other sounds. Om represents the four states of consciousness: waking, dreaming, sleeping, and transcendental, as well as the past, present and future. The Sanskrit symbol for Om comprises three separate Sanskrit letters and looks like ॐ.

The Upanishads teach that the mind is rooted in the heart and that to meditate on Om will lead you from your mind to your heart and from your heart to your divine soul. Om stands for the supreme Reality. It is a symbol for what was, what is, and what shall be. Om represents what lies beyond the past, present, and future. (Mandukya)

Taking some time to learn how to sing or chant Om and to feel its vibration is well worth the effort.

Begin by taking a comfortable sitting position and tune into your breath for a few minutes.

Place your hands over your sternum and breathe in fully. Open your mouth and let a long "aaaaahh" sound out as you exhale. Practice this several times and feel for the vibration of the "aaaaahh" beneath your hands. Repeat several times.

Cup your hands gently around your throat and breathe in fully. Open your mouth and let a long "ooooooo" sound (as in toe) out as you exhale. Practice this several times and feel for the vibration of the "ooooooo" beneath your hands. Repeat several times.

Place one hand at the back your head and the other on the crown of your head. Breathe in fully and let a long "mmmmmmm" sound out as you exhale. Practice this several times and feel for the vibration of the "mmmmmmm" beneath your hands. Repeat several times.

Experiment with letting your upper and lower teeth lightly rest against each other until you find the right amount of pressure that triggers bone resonance in your skull. Experiment and play around with different tones and pitches, as well as the placement of your tongue in your mouth, to notice if the vibrations can be felt more easily.

Now it's time to combine sounds. Merge the "aaaaahh" and the "ooooooo" until you get an "aahhooooo" sound. Feel for the movement of the vibration from your heart to your throat area. Finally add the "mmmmmmm," feeling the vibration go to the back of your head and finally out the crown of the head. Altogether it's "ahooommmm" or Om.

The Om offers a powerful balancing effect. Concentrate on the "O" if your goal is to balance the physical body. To do so, let the "O" last longer than the "M."

If your goal is for mental and spiritual balance, focus on the "M." Simply spend more time with the "M." This is especially effective as a prelude to meditation.

If you are interested in balancing the body with the mind and spirit, give equal time to the "O" and the "M."

Om can be used by itself. It is customary to sing it either once or in a series of three in a row. Let the sound flow with your breath in a free and easy manner. Om is the first word of many Sanskrit chants.

Singing or chanting Om is wonderful when done in chorus with a group of people. Encourage people to find their own pitch and to follow their own breath rate. In other words, people do not have to stay in unison. When the group Om ends, save time for a minute of silence to savor the effect.

Om Meditation

Guided Meditation

Time: Variable

Summary: Om can effectively be used as a mantra for meditation. Choose a mantra and practice it regularly. Notice the effects it has for you. After a while use a different one and feel what is unique to that mantra. From this process of experimentation and discovery, select one that resonates for you.

Here are some classical Sanskrit mantras that have been used for thousands of years by spiritual seekers and dedicated meditators.

Om

Hari Om — Purifies and removes obstacles and awakens the natural energy in the body. It is pronounced hah-ree om. (ree as in free)

Om Shanti Om Shanti Om — Shanti means peace and this mantra creates a peaceful feeling. It is pronounced Om SHAN-tee.

Om Namah Shivaya — I honor the God within myself and all others. (Om NAH-mah SHEE-vah-yah)

Sit in a comfortable, upright position and close your eyes. Focus your attention on your breath ... Breathe in softly and evenly ... in ... and out. Take time to allow your breath to focus your mind ... just focusing your mind on your breath ... when your mind begins to wander ... bring your attention back to your breath ... simply breathing in ... and out.

Begin to say Om (or any of the other mantras listed above) to yourself. You may synchronize it with your breathing or simply repeat it slowly, again and again.

Listen to the sound as you slowly repeat Om, again and again ... When your mind wanders ... bring your attention back to repeating the Om.

Allow your attention to focus more and more on the sound of Om ... Notice the qualities Om brings to your awareness ... allow your awareness to sink into the sound and space of Om ... immersing yourself in what Om reveals.

When your mind wanders, begin repeating Om, over and over, until your mind and awareness become still again ... slowly saying Om, over and over ... allow yourself to soak into the conscious awareness of Om.

Pause.

At some point, surround yourself ... immerse yourself into the awareness and space created by Om ... letting go of the need to repeat the Om ... hearing it echoing internally ... repeating itself.

Pause.

When your mind wanders, begin repeating Om, over and over, until your mind and awareness become still again ... Slowly saying Om, over and over ... allow yourself to soak into the conscious awareness of Om.

Pause.

Gradually, let go of mentally repeating Om and rest in the stillness.

When your mind wanders, begin repeating Om, over and over, until your mind and awareness become still again ... Slowly saying Om, over and over ... allow yourself to soak into the conscious awareness of Om.

Pause.

Slowly bring your awareness back to your breath and body ... become more and more aware of your surroundings ... When you're ready, open your eyes and sit quietly ... Gently stretch when you're ready.

Japa ~ Om Mantra Repetition

Mantra Repetition

Time: Variable

Summary: The repetition of a mantra is called japa. It can be repeated out loud, in a whisper, or silently. Some recommend repeating a mantra 108 times. A string of prayer beads, called a mala, can be used to keep your attention focused on the repetition of a mantra and to keep track of the number being said. Malas have from 27 to 108 beads. If a mala of 27 beads were used, it would be necessary to go around four times. A rosary can also be used as it has 54 beads. Simply go around twice, omitting the five beads at the crucifix.

There are thousands of mantras from which to choose. Mantras can be a sound, word, or phrase and can be in any language, although in yoga, they are commonly done in Sanskrit, from ancient India. Each mantra has its own signature vibration to discover. Several examples are given in the guided Om Meditation that precedes this description.

Mindfulness

Guided Meditation and Practice

Time: Mindfulness is being present in the moment. Once learned, it can be done in any situation and at any time. In the beginning, it is best learned through a regular daily practice. Start with five to ten minutes once or twice daily as a formal sitting practice and gradually increase over time. This will make it easier to remember to practice mindfulness at other times.

Summary: In a word, mindfulness is presence. It is the awareness of each immediate life-moment: awareness of feelings, sensations, thoughts, dreams, memories, opinions, moods, mental states, and emotions — without identifying with any of it as "who you are." "Mindfulness means paying attention in a particular way: on purpose, in the present moment, and nonjudgmentally," says Jon Kabat-Zinn. Doing so opens up an entirely new way of living and being by cultivating the ability to live more spaciously. By calming the mind, we are able to notice thinking as a mental activity and release identifying with our thoughts. This provides a safe haven from worries and fears associated with the past and future. The practice enables us to release fear, anger, or resistance to whatever is happening, allowing us instead to choose a compassionate response. The practice of mindfulness enables us to interact with daily life as a direct experience. It gives us a fresh vantage point from which to learn to trust in ourselves. Mindfulness practice also contends that if we can spaciously "hold" the moment, without grasping or avoiding, an inner knowing or higher truth will emerge and guide us to serve our best interest in harmony with the order of the Universe.

Although mindfulness meditation has its roots in Buddhism, it is helpful and constructive to people of any faith. If understanding and experience are to deepen our faith, we have to develop the ability to calm our mind and stay in the present moment, no matter what spiritual tradition we follow. In essence, we must move from belief into direct experience. Through meditation, writes Lama Surya Das, we come to know that "we are not what we think," rather we are the awareness that perceives the thoughts, knowing we are not the thoughts themselves. Even though we are responsible for our thoughts, it is important not to be limited by them. Going deeper into the moment uncovers our genuine being in our original, unprocessed, natural state. This is our true nature — boundless awareness that is at the heart of all of us. The Buddha described it as still, clear, lucid, empty, profound, simple (uncomplicated), and at peace.

Formal Mindfulness Meditation Techniques

Moment-to-moment awareness is cultivated in a formal meditation practice by learning to move beyond identifying and reacting to the thinking mind to focusing undivided attention on whatever is being experienced in the here and now.

Through being mindful of thoughts, feelings, perceptions, and sensations that occur, recognizing them with compassion, and letting them go as soon as they come up, we grow into a spacious awareness of our true self. One of the best ways to develop mindfulness is to be aware of your breath. Conscious breathing and Vipassana are two methods to get you started. Either method can be practiced well into the future and will bless you with the gifts inherent in living in the here and now.

Whichever technique is used, it is important to maintain an upright, erect posture because posture affects clarity of mind. Keep your eyes barely open or softly shut. The whole experience of the breath is very important; therefore, allow it to be spontaneous, natural, and effortless rather than regulated or forced. As always, begin each sitting meditation with a few minutes to still your body-mind.

Method One: Conscious Breathing means simply being aware of when you breathe in and when you breathe out, saying to yourself "Breathing in, I know I'm breathing in; breathing out, I know I'm breathing out," or if you like, shorten it to "in-out." This practice was originally taught by the Buddha. Thich Nhat Hahn, among others, brings these teachings to light today.

Method Two: Vipassana Meditation is practiced by focusing your awareness on one aspect of your breath. Select a place in your body as a vantage point from which to observe your breathing. This could be at the tip of the nostrils, the back of the throat, the upper chest, the middle chest, the belly, or the back. Try these various places in your body and choose whichever location gives you the easiest and most vivid contact with the sensations of breathing in and out. Let go of trying to control your breathing patterns, rhythms, or duration in any way and maintain your focus on your vantage point.

You will soon notice all sorts of things that distract you from watching your breath: some from inside you, some from the world around you. It may be a racing mind, restless limbs, a noisy truck, a barking dog, a pleasant memory, a creative thought, and all manner of mental impressions and feelings. In fact, mindfulness of the ongoing, endless activity of the mind is usually the first awareness of meditation. Luckily, the meditation tradition teaches that the mind doesn't have to behave this way and gives ways of training it to be focused and relaxed. So, as soon as you notice your meandering awareness, practice the art of naming. Instead of fighting, judging, or pushing away what is going on, lightly name what you have noticed with compassion and kindness and without judging, which is just another form of thinking. Name it thinking, hearing, perceiving, feeling emotions, bodily sensations, or whatever it is, and then return your awareness to your vantage point and find your breath. This is a practical way of being present with yourself. Although in the beginning, it may seem fruitless, after a while, mindfulness practice will give you mental relief, peace, and emotional space.

Informal Mindfulness: Throughout daily life, make a point of bringing your awareness into your breath when you might ordinarily be reactive, impatient, or fearful. For example, when you are stuck in traffic, instead of unconsciously practicing irritation, try mindful breathing as a way to relax into a larger, more spacious reality. How? When you notice you are compulsively or fearfully thinking about the past or future and unaware of this present moment, you can bring your attention to your vantage point, then your breath, and experientially return to who you really are. Likewise, your focal point may be whatever is taking place in the moment. In other words, only eat while you eat, only sleep while you sleep, and so on. Doing so sounds simple, but it is not easy. It will definitely be transformative.

Authors Note: Escaping into the safety of the present moment.

A few years ago, Angie, my Mom, was diagnosed with metastatic cancer, and the primary site could not be located. She had to undergo all sorts of undesirable procedures, causing her to be very weak and in pain a lot of the time. No known treatments were available because the primary site remained unidentified. Eventually, she regained her strength and went from being confined to a wheelchair to walking on her own. Miraculously and much to everyone's surprise and relief, her cancer tumor markers returned to the normal range and stayed there until the end. When asked, she smiled and said, "Honey, it's all in how you think and in all the love I'm getting." About a year later, she broke her hip in a fall, had surgery, and got a super-infection in the hospital. Along with medications, she was able to "out smart" the infection but was unable to overcome the effects of the surgery. She passed on several months later.

Luckily, my husband and I had just moved back home from living out of state, enabling me to take care of her during this time. The worries, fears, and emotions I felt could have easily engulfed me and torn me apart. Instead, living in the now was my salvation. I regularly practiced mindfulness in the moment, and it soon became my friend and ally. I thought of it as escaping into the safety of the present moment. Every day, my daily practice was to stay present and keep my heart open no matter what was happening and do my best to be in the experience without resistance. Resistance, I noticed, made everything feel much worse. This opened me up to many laughs and joyful times as well as to anger and despair. It enabled me to enjoy my mother's company and be attentive to her needs while I was with her. She often said, "Julie, honey, you know what I need before I do!" This was because I remained watchful and was able to anticipate what she needed. Rather than dwelling on and carrying with me the gravity of these circumstances when I was away from her, I practiced being in that here and now. I did this by enjoying the sunshine, springtime, my other activities, and most of all my family and friends. Whenever I found myself caught up in fear and other feelings not based on the present, I returned to what was present and went with that. Believe me, it wasn't easy, but it helped tremendously. Honestly, many times, the present moment offered me the only way into peace and pleasure in the midst of misery.

In due course, the heartache subsided, and as I continued to practice formal and informal mindfulness, the tide eventually turned from grief to gratitude. Personally, teaching and practicing hatha yoga is an enormous source of moment-to-moment awareness for me. It gives me a lot of joy.

A few years later, my beloved younger brother, Tommy, died unexpectedly after a five-day stay in the hospital. My grief was strong and overwhelming. My husband and friends blanketed me with love and support all throughout this time, and once again, mindfulness and prayers pulled me through. My heartbreaking sadness seemed constant for quite a while, but whenever it hit me, I turned my attention to whatever I was experiencing physically in the moment. This was usually a pounding, heavy heart, a sick feeling in my gut, and burning hot tears. The instant I did this, the raging emotions immediately and significantly lessened. It was quite noticeable that my thinking mind was fueling my emotions, and if I let go of resistance and focused on the present, instead of allowing my mind to dwell in the past or the future, the wave of emotion would pass. Meditation allowed me to be more in touch with my feelings without being driven or controlled by them. Eckhart Tolle calls it "awareness without thinking" in his book *The Power of Now*. Being present-minded during this time also allowed me to witness coincidences and occurrences that were truly miraculous. Each and every time this happened, comfort poured into my being. What a Godsend.

I urge you to cultivate the art of mindfulness. Living will take on a remarkable depth of meaning. Your heart and soul will be touched.

Walking Meditation

Yoga Practice

Contributed by Charles MacInerney

Time: 15 to 60 minutes

Walking Meditation is easy to practice and enhances physical, mental, and spiritual well-being. Beginners will find it to be a wonderful initiation into the art of meditation, and seasoned meditators will appreciate all the advantages of the practice, as well as the opportunity for a moving meditation. It is especially effective for those who find it difficult to sit still for long periods of time.

In response to inclement weather or a desire for privacy, some people prefer to practice indoors by walking around the perimeter of a large room. Others enjoy practicing outdoors in their yard or in a beautiful outdoor setting, like a park. If you practice outdoors, choose a scenic and quiet setting. Walk without a destination. Typically, we are always going somewhere when we walk. Even in the park, we tend to plan out our walk. "I will walk down to the picnic tables, around the duck pond, and return to my car". Then, as we walk, we constantly measure how far we have come or how far we have left to walk, and our mind dwells on the past or the future. Instead, wander aimlessly without arriving, being somewhere rather than going somewhere, dwelling in the present moment.

Walking meditation should generally be practiced for 15 minutes to an hour. A 5- to 20-minute walking meditation can also be used as a break between two 20-minute sitting meditations. This allows a longer period for meditation without placing undue physical demands on the body. Furthermore, it helps with making the transition from sitting meditation to being able to be meditative while in motion.

At the start, begin walking a little faster than normal, then gradually slow down to a normal walking speed, continuing to slow down even more until you start to feel off balance or unnatural. Speed up just enough to feel comfortable, physically and psychologically. At first you may need to walk fairly fast to feel smooth in your gait, but with practice, as your balance improves, you should be able to walk more slowly. Please note that you do not have to walk slowly. In fact, you can apply these same practices to running, thus converting jogging into a meditative experience.

Be mindful of your breathing, without trying to control it. It is preferable if you can freely breathe in and out through your nose, but if you struggle with nasal breathing, it is okay to breathe through your mouth. Allow your breath to become deep and diaphragmatic, if possible, but always make sure your breathing feels natural, not artificial. Allow your breath to become circular and fluid.

Walk with "soft vision" allowing your eyes to relax and focus upon nothing, while aware of everything. Smile softly with your eyes. Gradually allow the smile to spread from your eyes to your face and throughout your body. This is called an "organic smile" or a "thalamus smile." Imagine every cell of your body smiling softly. Let all worry and sadness fall away from you as you walk.

Be mindful of your walking, making each step a gesture so you move in a state of grace, leaving each footprint as an impression of the peace and love you feel for the universe. Walk with slow, small, deliberate, balanced, graceful footsteps, being aware of the motions with each step along the way. Walk in silence, both internally and externally.

After a while, when both your breath and your walking have slipped into a regular pattern of their own accord, become aware of the number of footsteps per breath. Make no effort to change your breath; rather lengthen or shorten the rhythm of your step just enough so that you have two, three, or four steps per inhalation and two, three, or four steps per exhalation. Once you have discovered your natural rhythm, lock into it so the rhythm of walking sets the rhythm for breathing like a metronome.

After several weeks of regular practice, you may experiment with the ratios — adding a footstep to your exhalation and later to your inhalation as well. Whatever ratio of steps-to-breath that you settle on, it should feel comfortable, and you should be able to maintain it comfortably for the duration of the meditation. After several months, you may find your lung capacity improving. If you are comfortable doing so, lengthen your breath an extra step, but avoid trying to slow your breath too much, or you will do more harm than good.

Notice the beauty of your surroundings, both externally and internally. Smile with every cell in your body.

Author's note: Charles MacInerney has practiced yoga since 1971. He teaches in Austin, Texas, and leads yoga retreats around the world. He is the founder of www.yogateacher.com and publishes the newsletter *Expanding Paradigms*. Charles is cofounder of the Texas Yoga Retreat and also of the Living Yoga Teacher Training Program. He is registered with Yoga Alliance at the 500 hr. level and regularly presents at national and international conferences. Charles has been interviewed for a variety of articles in *Yoga Journal* in addition to writing their "Ask the Expert" column in June of 2004. He also appeared in the *Wall Street Journal.*

Timeless Treasures:
Reflecting and Contemplating
on the Wisdom of Yoga

The meditations and reflections that follow answer the age-old questions: "Who am I? What is my true nature? What is my purpose? How do I handle obstacles and suffering? and What gifts come from living within the path of yoga?" The insights that follow are from the perspective of yoga's wisdom teachings, which originated over 5000 years ago in India. Originally, these teachings were revealed to yogis in meditation when their hearts and souls became unified with and established in the oneness of the universal intelligence. Their students then memorized and orally passed this wisdom down from generation to generation until they were written down in Sanskrit.

The lessons that follow come from English translations of the Upanishads, Bhagavad-Gita, and the Yoga Sutras of Patanjali. I have studied several translations of the texts listed in the bibliography. Each author translates the original Sanskrit sources using slightly different words. I have reworded and reordered them to aid my understanding and hopefully yours. The meditations that follow capture my current understanding — the process is evolutionary. I am grateful to the authors of these texts and take respon- sibility if my interpretations are misleading in any way. I am continually amazed at how wise and relevant this work is in my life today, and it is my hope that you will investigate these profound works on your own for inspi- ration and to discover guidance and insights for living a spirit-filled life.

As in the traditional way, it is recommended that the following teachings be listened to and reflected on as they are read aloud. Reading them silently and contemplating each of them will be helpful as well. Perhaps meditate on a new one each day. The Upanishads teach over and over again that true understanding comes from the experience of living and breathing these lessons on a daily basis. So please, take the teachings from these writings into your life by finding your own personal way of doing so.

Yoga's wisdom on one's true nature

Love is the first seed of the Soul.   Rig Veda x.29

Our essential nature is boundless consciousness.
    We are rooted in it when the mind focuses and settles.
                                        Yoga Sutra 1.3
For the soul there is neither birth nor death.
    The soul that is will never cease to be.
    It is unborn, eternal, ever existing, undying, and primeval.
    One's essence does not die when the body dies.
                                        Bhagavad Gita 2.20
There is a spirit which is pure and
    which is beyond old age and death;
    and beyond hunger and thirst and sorrow.
    This is Atman, one's Spirit.
    All desires of this Spirit are Truth.
    It is this Spirit that we must find and know.
                                        Chandogya Upanishad

Being on the yoga path

You alone can walk the inner path.   Upanishads

Many paths are possible;
    whichever path is sincerely traveled
    leads to inner peace.   Bhagavad Gita 4.11

Whichever path you follow will lead to divine love in the end.
    Your love will be returned with divine love.
                                        Bhagavad Gita 4.1
It is better to follow your own life purpose poorly,
    than to do another's perfectly.
    You are safe from harm
    when you follow your own unique path.   Bhagavad Gita 3.35

Do not give up your own natural life path, even though it is flawed;
    all actions contain flaws, as fire is surrounded by smoke.
                                        Bhagavad Gita 18.48
No effort is wasted and no gain is ever lost when on this path;
    even a little practice will shelter you from sorrow and
    protect you from the greatest fear.   Bhagavad Gita 2.40

The meanings and practice of yoga

The practice of yoga is to
  become established in the state of freedom and
  peace of mind.   Yoga Sutra 1.13

Yoga is the settling of the mind into stillness. Yoga Sutra 1.2

Yoga is equanimity of mind.   Bhagavad Gita 2.48

Yoga is skill in actions without regard for results.
                                              Bhagavad Gita 2.50

Karma Yoga / Selfless Service

Perform all actions
  with no attachment to results and
  in the spirit of devotion.
  Control of the senses and
  using them in selfless service
  is the yoga of action.   Bhagavad Gita 3.9, 3.7

Act for the sake of action.
  Do not be inactive.   Bhagavad Gita 2.47

The wise person is impartial to all results,
  whether good or bad, and
  focuses on the action alone.   Bhagavad Gita 2.50

The divine is indifferent to results.   Bhagavad Gita 4.14

The yoga of *action* is the path and tranquility results.
                                              Bhagavad Gita 6.3

Jnana Yoga / Knowledge and Wisdom

Nothing in the world can purify
    as powerfully as spiritual knowledge and wisdom.
    You will find this wisdom within yourself
    on this path of yoga.   Bhagavad Gita 4.38

Bhakti Yoga / Love and Devotion

Devotion, perfect faith and belief in the One is a superior path.
                                 Bhagavad Gita 6.47

No matter what name is used,
    those devoted to God
    are really worshipping the One,
    even if they don't know it.   Bhagavad Gita 9.23

Raja Yoga / Meditation

The essence of yoga is
    when your mind is undisturbed and
    is absorbed in deep meditation.
    This equanimity is the essence of yoga.   Bhagavad Gita 2.53

When the five senses and the mind are still,
    and reason itself rests in silence,
    then begins the path supreme.
    This calm steadiness of the senses is called yoga.
                             Katha Upanishad

Hatha Yoga / Yoga Asanas and Pranayama
(yoga postures and breathing)

The physical postures of yoga should be steady and comfortable.
Yoga Sutra 2.46

Physical postures are mastered
    when practiced mindfully, effortlessly,
    and with awareness of the Infinite.   Yoga Sutra 2.47

The breathing practices stabilize
    and balance the flow of breath
    and increase life energy.   Yoga Sutra 2.49

Controlling the volume, duration, and frequency
    of the inhalation, the exhalation,
    and the pauses between each breath,
    refines and slows the breathing.
    This enhances prana,
    the energy that supports and sustains the life force.
Yoga Sutra 2.50

Yoga's wisdom on the mind

The mind becomes peaceful and free
    when the qualities of the heart are cultivated:
    friendship toward the joyful,
    compassion toward the suffering,
    happiness toward the pure, and
    indifference toward the impure.   Yoga Sutra 1.33

The mind is the best of friends
    for the person who has mastered it.
    The mind is a sly opponent
    for those who have not.   Bhagavad Gita 6.6

Concentrating the whole mind on a single object
    will soon purify it.   Bhagavad Gita 6.12

The mind is hard to master, but it can be done
    if you keep striving earnestly and in the right direction.
        Bhagavad Gita 6.36

When disturbed by negative thoughts and feelings,
    cultivate the opposite.   Yoga Sutra 2.33

The senses are superior and stronger than matter;
    mind is higher and stronger than the senses;
    and higher and stronger than the mind is intelligence;
    but the highest and strongest of all is the soul.
        Bhagavad Gita 3.42

Our essential nature is usually overshadowed by mental activity.
    The five types of mental activity are
    understanding, misunderstanding, imagination, sleep and memory.
    They may or may not cause suffering.   Yoga Sutra 1.4-6

The five causes of suffering are
    ignorance of our real nature, egoism,
    attachment, aversion, and fear, especially of death.
        Yoga Sutra 2.3

Obstacles to mental clarity are illness, fatigue, doubt,
    carelessness, idleness, dullness, attachment, illusion,
    overindulgence, lack of perseverance, and regression.

                                         Yoga Sutra 1.30

These distractions make the body restless,
    the breathing unsteady, agitate the mind,
    and cause stress.   Yoga Sutra 1.31

Freedom from the influence of desire and cravings
    constitutes self-mastery.
    The mind no longer longs for anything it has seen or heard of;
    even what is promised in the scriptures.   Yoga Sutra 1.15

Yoga's tenets of life and living

Yamas, or the tenets of life from the Yoga Sutras, are
  Reverence for all life,
  Truthfulness,
  Integrity,
  Moderation, and
  Nonattachment.   Yoga Sutra 2.30

Niyamas, or the tenets for living from the Yoga Sutras, are
  Purity,
  Contentment,
  Discipline,
  Self-understanding, and
  Surrender to the Lord   Yoga Sutra 2.32

Whatever a great person does
  will set the standards for others to follow.
                                              Bhagavad Gita 3.21

The wise person does not disturb the minds of the ignorant.
  Instead, the wise person inspires others by quietly acting
  in the spirit of yoga.
                                              Bhagavad Gita 3.26

There is a path of joy and a path of pleasure.
  Both are attractive.
  The wise choose everlasting joy;
  fools choose temporary pleasure.
                                              Katha Upanishads 1.30

Practicing the yoga way of life

Where there is creation there is joy.
    There is no joy in the finite.
    Joy is only in the Infinite:
    Know the nature of the Infinite.   Chandogya Upanishad.

Future pain should be prevented.   Yoga Sutra 2.16

Yoga will destroy all suffering for the person who is
    moderate in food and pleasure,
    moderate in action,
    moderate in sleep and waking.   Bhagavad Gita 6.17

When we are firmly established in moderation,
    subtle energy is generated.   Yoga Sutra 2.38

When we are firmly established in nonviolence,
    all beings around cease being hostile.   Yoga Sutra 2.35

When we are firmly established in truthfulness and honesty,
    success automatically follows.   Yoga Sutra 2.36

When nonattachment is established,
    the nature and purpose of life is understood.
                                              Yoga Sutra 2.39

Just like a well is unnecessary to a village on the banks of a river,
    the scriptures are unnecessary to the person who knows the truth.
                                              Bhagavad Gita 2.4

The practice of yoga will be firmly grounded
    when it is maintained consistently
    and with dedication over a long time.
                                              Yoga Sutra 1.14

Yoga Blessings

Om asa toma sat gamaya

Tamaso ma jyotir gamaya

Mrityor ma amritam gamaya

Om shanti, shanti, shanti

Lead us from the unreal to the Real

Lead us from darkness to the Light

Lead us from the fear of death to the

Knowledge of immortality

Om peace, peace, peace

      Brihad-Aranyaka Upanishad 1.3.28

Universal Prayer

Loka samasta sukino bhavantu

May the entire universe be filled with peace and joy, love and light.

Resources and Bibliography

Breathing Resources

Farhi, Donna., *The Breathing Book: Good Health and Vitality Through Essential Breath Work*. New York: Henry Holt and Company, 1996.

Chakra Resources

Judith, Anodea, *Chakra Balancing*. Boulder, CO: Sounds True, 2003.

Judith, Anodea, *Eastern Body, Western Mind: Psychology and the Chakra System*, Berkeley, CA: Celestial Arts Publishing, 1996.

Judith, Anodea, *Wheels of Life: A Users Guide to the Chakra System*, St. Paul, MN: Llewellyn Publications, 2001.

Guided Imagery Resources

Achterberg, Dossey, Kolkmeier, *Rituals of Healing: Using Imagery for Health and Wellness*. New York, NY. Bantam Books, 1994.

Lusk, Julie T., *30 Scripts for Relaxation, Imagery and Inner Healing, Vols. One and Two*. Duluth, MN: Whole Person Press, 1992, 1993.

Naparstek, Belleruth. *Staying Well with Guided Imagery*. New York, NY: Warner Books, 1994.

Naparstek, Belleruth at www.healthjourneys.com

Guided Relaxation Recordings

Lusk, Julie T.,

   Wholesome Energizers, Cincinnati, OH: Card*plus*CD. 2004

   Wholesome Relaxation, Cincinnati, OH: Card*plus*CD. 2003

   Refreshing Journeys, Duluth, MN: Whole Person Associates. 1995

Naparstek, Belleruth. HealthJourneys.com

Whole Person Associates Recordings. 800-247-6789

Meditation Resources

Durgananda, Swami (Sally Kempton). *The Heart of Meditation: Pathways to a Deeper Experience*. S. Fallsburg, NY. SYDA Foundation, 2002.

Keating, Thomas., *Open Mind, Open Heart*. New York, NY: Continuim Publishing Co. 1986, 1982.

Kornfield, Jack. *Meditation for Beginners*. Boulder, CO: Sounds True, 2004.

Music

Card*plus*CD Music by Tom Laskey 800-700-9265

New Earth Records 800-570-4074

Whole Person Associates 800-247-6789

Yoga Practice Books

Anderson, S., Sovik, R. *Yoga, Mastering the Basics*. Honesdale, PA, Himalayan Ins., 2000.

Baxter, Christopher, *Kripalu Hatha Yoga*, Lenox, MA, Kripalu Center for Yoga. 1998.

Carrico, Mara. *Yoga Journal's Yoga Basics*. NY, NY, Henry Holt, 1997.

Devi, Nischala. *The Healing Path of Yoga*. NY, NY, Three Rivers Press. 2000.

Folan, Lilias. *Lilias! Yoga Gets Better with Age*. Emmaus, PA, Rodale, 2005.

Folan, Lilias. *Lilias, Yoga & Your Life*. New York: Collier Books, 1981.

Lasater, Judith. *Relax and Renew*. Berkeley, CA, Rodmell Press. 1995.

Lusk, Julie. *Desktop Yoga* ™. NY, NY, Perigee Press. 1998.

Muktibodhananda, Swami. *Hatha Yoga Pradipika*. Bihar India, Bihar School of Yoga, 1985, 1993.

Scarvelli, Vanda. *Awakening the Spine*. San Francisco. CA, Harper, 1991.

Van Lysebeth, Andre. *Yoga Self-Taught*. New York: Barnes & Noble, 1971.

Yoga Practice Videos and DVDs

Folan, Lilias

    Go to naturaljourneys.com for all of Lilias's products

Friend, John

    Anusara Yoga Essentials (audio)

    Yoga for Meditators

Ward, Susan Winter.

    Embracing Menopause. 1998

    Yoga for the Young at Heart. 1998

White and Rich.

    Flow Series. White Lotus Foundation.

    Total Yoga. White Lotus Foundation.

Yoga Journal's: Healing Arts Series:

    For Beginners

    For Energy

    For Strength

    For Relaxation

    For Flexibility

    Prenatal Yoga

Books on Yogis

Dass, Ram, *Miracle of Love: Stories about Neem Karoli Baba;* Santa Fe, NM, 1979, 1995.

Levitt, Jo Ann, *Pilgrim of Love: The Life and Teachings of Swami Kripalu;* Consortium, 2004.

Yogananda, Paramahansa, *Autobiography of a Yogi,* SRF, Los Angeles, CA, 1973.

Yoga Philosophy and Inspiration

Feuerstein, Georg. *Shambhala Encyclopedia of Yoga*. Boston, MA, Shambhala Publications, Inc. 1997.

Faulds, Danna. *Go In and In: Poems from the Heart of Yoga.* Peaceable Kingdom Books, Greenville, VA, 2002.

———— *One Soul: More Poems from the Heart of Yoga.* Peaceable Kingdom Books, Greenville, VA, 2003.

———— *Prayers to the Infinite: New Yoga Poems.* Peaceable Kingdom Books, Greenville, VA, 2004.

The Upanishads

Easwaran, Eknath. *The Upanishads,* Translated for the Modern Reader. USA: Nilgiri Press, 1987.

Mascaro, Juan. *The Upanishads.* New York: Penguin, 1965.

Shearer, Alistair. *The Upanishads.* New York: Bell Tower, 1978.

The Yoga Sutras

Desikachar, T. K. V. *The Heart of Yoga, Developing a Personal Practice.* Rochester, VT: Inner Traditions International, 1995.

Satchidananda, Sri Swami. *The Yoga Sutras of Patanjali.* Yogaville, VA: Integral Yoga Publications, 1990.

Shearer, Alistair. *The Yoga Sutras of Patanjali.* New York: Bell Tower, 1982.

Bhagavad Gita

Mitchell, Stephen. *Bhagavad Gita, a New Translation.* New York: Harmony Books, 2000.

Satchidananda, Sri Swami. *The Living Gita.* New York: Henry Holt and Company, 1988.

Stoler Miller, Barbara. *The Bhagavad Gita.* Quality Paperback Book Club, 1998.

Inspirational Resources

Read the Bible, Tao Te Ching and writings by or about the Buddha, Kabir, Rumi, Hafiz, Thich Nhat Hanh, and Ram Dass

Julie T. Lusk, M.Ed.

http://wholesomeresources.com

JuLusk@aol.com
C/O Whole Person Associates
210 West Michigan
Duluth, MN 55802-1908
800-247-6789

Julie Lusk, M.Ed., is president of Wholesome Resources, an internationally renowned author, and a dynamic and inspiring speaker. Julie has over 25 years of expertise in stress management, wellness, yoga, and guided imagery. Professionally, Julie has worked in health care management, higher education and community organizing. Thousands have benefited from her volunteer work.

Julie's other publications include:

Books

30 Scripts for Relaxation, Imagery and Inner Healing, Volume One
Whole Person Associates, Duluth, MN 800-247-6789

30 Scripts for Relaxation, Imagery and Inner Healing, Volume Two
Whole Person Associates, Duluth, MN 800-247-6789

Desktop Yoga ™ *The Anywhere, Anytime Relaxation Program*
Perigee/Penguin/Putnam Books, New York, NY

Relaxation Recordings

Refreshing Journeys (Recorded relaxation sampler from 30 Scripts)
Whole Person Associates, Duluth, MN 800-247-6789

Wholesome Relaxation
Wholesome Energizers
Card*plus*CD, Cincinnati, OH 800-700-9265

CPSIA information can be obtained at www.ICGtesting.com
Printed in the USA
BVOW04s0022281014

372604BV00001B/3/A